MAKING WISE MEDICAL DECISIONS

How to Get the Information You Need

Resources for Rehabilitation
Lexington, Massachusetts

Resources for Rehabilitation
33 Bedford Street, Suite 19A
Lexington, MA 02420
(781) 862-6455
FAX (781) 861-7517
e-mail: info@rfr.org   www.rfr.org

Making Wise Medical Decisions: How to Get the Information You Need

ISBN 0-929718-29-1

Library of Congress Cataloging-in-Publication Data

Making Wise Medical Decisions: How to Get the Information You Need--2nd edition
   p.   cm.
Includes bibliographical references and index.
ISBN 0-929718-29-1 (pbk.   : alk.paper)
1. Health--Decision-making--Popular works. 2. Medicine--Decision-making--Popular works. 3. Medicine--Information services--Popular works. 4. Physician services utilization--Popular works. 5. Consumer education. I. Resources for Rehabilitation (Organization)

RA776.5.M266   2001
362.1--dc21   2001041668
                                                     CIP

For a complete listing of publications available from Resources for Rehabilitation, see pages 252-256

TABLE OF CONTENTS

ORGANIZATION OF THIS BOOK

This book is designed to help medical consumers and their family members or other caregivers locate information that helps them to make wise, rational decisions regarding health care. It provides information to help develop a strategy for seeking out information and guides readers to sources of information on a variety of topics related to health care.

In addition to extensive narrative information, each chapter includes annotated listings about organizations, publications, and tapes that may contribute to making wise medical decisions; they are listed alphabetically within chapters. Although many of the publications described are available in libraries or bookstores, the addresses and phone numbers of publishers and distributors are included for those who wish to purchase the books by mail, phone, or online. Some books that are out of print are included; these may be located in libraries or bookstores that specialize in locating out of print books.

Developments in computer technology, such as the Internet and e-mail, have greatly increased access to information about health issues for the general public. Internet and e-mail addresses are included when available. Most web sites begin with "www" (which stands for world wide web), but some do not have this as part of their addresses.

All of the material is up-to-date, and prices were accurate at the time of publication. However, it is always advisable to contact publishers to inquire about availability and current prices. Very frequently, businesses, especially publishers, merge, changing their names, addresses, and web sites. It is very difficult to keep abreast of these changes, but often their toll-free numbers remain the same. Alternatively, entering the organization's name into a search engine on the Internet (such as yahoo.com) may result in locating the current web site.

The phone numbers of organizations that have special telephone access for people with hearing or speech impairments, formerly called telecommunications devices for the deaf (TDD), are now called text telephones (TT). When organizations have these special devices, the phone number is followed by the notation "(TT)." When the same number is available for either voice or text telephone access, "(V/TT)" appears after the phone number. FAX numbers are also included when available. Phone numbers that begin with either (800), (866), (877), or (888) are toll-free.

Since telephone area codes have been changing frequently, if you experience difficulty in reaching the number listed, check the area code of the organization you are calling.

WHY THIS BOOK WAS WRITTEN

Two contemporary, complementary trends have served as the inspiration for writing this book. First, many individuals who use the health care system (and who doesn't?) have come to realize that it is important to be active participants in decisions regarding their own medical treatment. Historically, consumers of medical care did not question the advice of physicians regarding medical treatment. In the traditional, professional model of medicine, the physician instructed the patient concerning medical treatment, and the patient accepted this advice without question. Although patients did not always comply with their doctors' advice, their reasons for failing to do so may have had more to do with the incompatibility of the advice with their lifestyle or fear of the recommended procedure than questioning the physician. Today, the situation has changed. According to a government study, "Today's consumers are demanding more -- and more detailed -- health information and are taking a more active role in making medical and lifestyle decisions" (General Accounting Office: 1996).

Second, there has been an explosion of medical information that is readily available to the public. Increased access to the Internet has made a broad range of medical information available at the click of a button. From medical journals to consumer support groups to professional medical societies and voluntary organizations, the wealth of health related information available on the Internet seems unlimited.

While increased access to information enables medical consumers to make more informed decisions, it is often difficult to locate this information efficiently. When medical conditions arise, both the affected individual and his or her family are under stress and may have difficulty locating the information they need in a timely manner. This book aims to eliminate the confusion and to direct medical consumers to find the information that answers their questions.

Significant numbers of individuals have indicated that they are not satisfied with the information that health care professionals provide. A study by the Picker Institute (Pham: 1997) found that 28% of the nearly 24,000 respondents felt that doctors' offices and clinics did not provide enough information, 31% were not told about side effects of prescribed medication, and 36% did not have enough say about their own treatment. A study (Braddock et al.: 1999) of patients' encounters with primary care physicians and surgeons found that very few (9%) medical decisions (including medical tests, medicine prescriptions, and procedures) were completely discussed. Another study found that patients who visited physicians who exhibited less participatory style were less satisfied and more likely to change physicians (Kaplan et al.: 1996). On the other hand, patients who receive more information were more satisfied with their medical encounters (Roter and Hall: 1992).

To compensate for these deficiencies, many patients have adopted a "consumerist" stance toward medical treatment (Haug and Lavin: 1981). Just as they question the quality of commodities that they purchase, many individuals in need of health care question their doctors' advice through second (and third) opinions and through reading about the recommended procedures themselves. With increasing specialization in the medical profession, medical consumers must be able to determine which medical treatment is best for them when different physicians proffer different opinions. Advances in high technology medical procedures require consumers to face the enormous task of filtering the information and locating what is pertinent to their specific case. This book was written to help individuals in this situation locate appropriate information without taking extraneous steps and time.

Studies over the past decades have found that individuals who have higher levels of participation in making medical decisions have better health outcomes than patients who have lower participation rates. Kaplan and her colleagues (1989), studying patients with chronic conditions such as diabetes and hypertension, found that those who asked more questions during physician visits, made more attempts to direct the conversation, and attempted to control the physician's behavior reported fewer lost work days, fewer health complaints, and fewer functional limitations due to their illness. When medical consumers ask more questions and receive more information from the physician, they are likely to have better health. Greenfield and his colleagues (1988) found that individuals with diabetes who, prior to their physician visit, were encouraged to ask questions, not only asked more questions of their physician than the control group who had no such training, but also had better control of their blood glucose (Also see, Schulman: 1979).

Not all physicians readily accept the role of patients as decision-makers. When physicians hold a monopoly over information, they retain their power over patients. Once patients become empowered with information, physicians lose their monopoly and often feel threatened (Haug: 1994). Patients wonder whether to pursue the course of asking questions, because if their physicians become angry, perhaps the patients will not receive the quality of medical care they need.

Finding a physician that encourages and cooperates in the medical consumer's search for information is critical to obtaining the best medical care. Perhaps physicians should take the attitude expressed by the sign on a reference librarian's desk, "There is no such thing as a dumb question. Please ask me."

References

Braddock, Clarence H. III et al.
1999   "Informed Decision Making in Outpatient Practice: Time to Get Back to Basics" JAMA 282(December 22-29):2313-2320
General Accounting Office
1996   Consumer Health Infomatics: Emerging Issues Washington DC: GAO/AIMD-96-86
Greenfield, Sheldon et al.
1988   "Patients' Participation in Medical Care: Effects on Blood Sugar Control and Quality of Life in Diabetes" Journal of General Internal Medicine 3(September/October):448-457
Haug, Marie
1994   "Elderly Patients, Caregivers, and Physicians: Theory and Research on Health Care Triads" Journal of Health and Social Behavior 35(March):1-12

Haug, Marie and Bebe Lavin
1981   "Practitioner or Patient - Who's in Charge?" <u>Journal of Health and Social Behavior</u> 22(September):212-229

Kaplan, S.H. et al.
1996   "Characteristics of Physicians with Participatory Decision-Making" <u>Annals of Internal Medicine</u> 124:5(March 1):497-504

Kaplan, Sherrie H., Sheldon Greenfield, and John E. Ware
1989   "Assessing the Effects of Physician-Patient Interactions on the Outcomes of Chronic Disease" <u>Medical Care</u> 27:3(Supplement):S110-S127

Pham, Alex
1997   "Health Survey: Patients Seek More Information, Input" <u>Boston Globe</u> January 28

Roter, Debra L. and Judith A. Hall
1992   <u>Doctors Talking with Patients, Patients Talking with Doctors</u> Westport, CT: Auburn House

Schulman, Beryl A.
1979   "Active Patient Orientation and Outcomes in Hypertension Treatment" <u>Medical Care</u> XVII:3:267-279

Chapter 1

GETTING THE INFORMATION YOU NEED
TO MAKE WISE MEDICAL DECISIONS

Obtaining the information that you need to make a wise medical decision often entails a multifaceted approach, including reviews of medical literature, discussions with a variety of medical personnel, and discussions with other medical consumers. When a medical problem occurs, obviously the first step is to seek out an evaluation from a physician. Following an examination, the physician should sit down with you and discuss the condition, its likely effects and prognosis, and options for treatment. You should ask as many appropriate questions as possible, but you should also schedule a follow-up visit, so that you have time to organize your thoughts and questions. In between visits, you should read about the condition and talk to others who have experienced it. Ask the physician to recommend articles on the condition and treatments. In cases of emergency, this strategy will not apply, but if the condition allows you any leeway to search out second opinions, review medical research, or have discussions with other medical consumers, you should pursue this course immediately.

Many physicians underestimate the amount of information that patients want. In a study of patients with hypertension (Strull et al.: 1984), 41% of patients wanted more information, and 29% of physicians underestimated the amount of information that patients wanted. In a study in which 69 general internists and 485 of their patients were asked to rank the importance of various aspects of health care, physicians and patients generally agreed on the importance of the physicians' clinical competence (Laine: 1994). Their greatest disagreement occurred in the area of communicating information. Communication about risks and benefits of treatment, answering patients' questions in an understandable way, presenting the diagnosis clearly, and discussing the purpose of taking drugs and instructions for their optimal use were ranked as highly important by patients, but physicians placed the importance of these issues far lower down on their rankings.

In a review of studies of physician-patient communication, Roter and Hall (1989) concluded that of all the patient variables studied, the amount of information provided by the health care professional was most likely to predict patient satisfaction. Yet physicians often feel threatened by the questions their patients ask, fearing a loss of power in the physician-patient relationship if they provide much information. By withholding information, physicians attempt to retain their dominant position in the relationship.

Learning about their medical conditions and the tests that are used to reach a diagnosis and treatment plan is particularly important for medical consumers who belong to managed care plans. Some of these plans have "gag" policies that prohibit physicians from discussing alternative treatment options that the particular plan does not provide because they are too expensive. Many states prohibit such "gag" policies; check with the state agency that licenses health care facilities to see if your state has passed such regulatory or legislative measures.

It is wise to plan a strategy for obtaining the information necessary for assessing your condition and treatment options. In most cases, the strategy will include visiting one or more libraries to obtain articles from medical journals and popular health magazines, using online resources to locate and obtain information, and speaking with others who are in a similar situation.

Keep records of all the places you have searched and the main points you have learned. Make a list of questions that develop as you go along to ask your physician. If your physician is unfamiliar with what you have read, provide a copy of the articles or references so that he or she may research the topic also.

THE LIBRARY

Medical school and hospital libraries are often open to the public; if no medical library is available, the local public library or a college or university library may have medical journals in their collections. If the library does not provide access to MEDLINE, (see "ONLINE RESOURCES" section below), ask the librarian for a referral to a library that does provide it. Look up your condition; you will find articles and the journals in which they appear. Then search the library's catalogue of holdings, now computerized in most libraries, to determine if any books have been written on the condition. Although some books may be available on the specific condition you are researching, sometimes it is necessary to search under a broader topic to find an appropriate publication. For example, books have been written on cataract surgery, since it is such a common procedure, but in order to find books that contain information on less common topics such as optic neuritis, it may be necessary to search under the topic "eye diseases." Both articles and books that are unavailable in the library you are using may be obtained by interlibrary loan. Ask the reference librarian for assistance.

In addition to the computerized catalogue, many libraries offer databases in which you can search for articles in current periodicals and for community information and referral. Info Trac is a popular database of periodical literature that includes both popular magazines and well known journals such as JAMA (Journal of the American Medical Association). You may search Info Trac by subject or keyword. For example, if you choose "diagnostic tests, noninvasive" as your subject, the database will search for articles which appeared in medical journals and popular publications within a specified time period and list them on the screen. Many of the articles will be available in abstract form, and some may be available in their entirety. The results may be downloaded to disk or printed out. Many libraries also offer a Community Information and Referral database that allows you to search by "agency" or "subject." This is especially helpful when you do not know the name of an organization. The reference librarian can demonstrate how to use these and other databases.

Many medical reference books are not only voluminous, but also rather expensive for the average consumer. Books such as the Directory of Physicians in the United States are often available in the reference section of public libraries, college or university libraries, and medical libraries. There is a voluntary organization for virtually every medical condition, even the most obscure. These may be listed in the Encyclopedia of Associations, found in the reference sections of most libraries. This reference work lists voluntary organizations by topic. Along with the descriptions of the organizations are addresses and phone numbers for their main offices. Many of these organizations have state and local chapters which conduct meetings to provide information and enable members to exchange information about their experiences and solutions to their common problems. These voluntary organizations also publish brochures, magazines, and books about the condition they specialize in. Although much of this information is very basic, it may lead you to terms and articles that you want to seek out for further information.

Articles on health and medical care are often found in popular magazines. Guides to periodical literature, located in the reference section of public libraries, index articles by topic. Most major newspapers devote space to health and medical reports. These reports describe new medical diagnostic tools, treatments, and resources. They may list national organizations, local support groups, and sources of adaptive technology. The newspaper may have a web site with an archive of these articles. Read articles about medical care that appear in the popular press with caution. Although well intended, these articles often tout new treatments that have not yet been adequately tested. For example, an article in the Boston Globe (Foreman: 1998) was devoted to two new techniques to help women with blood disorders and uterine fibroids that caused excessive menstrual bleeding. The article described two women who each had undergone one of the techniques and endorsed these treatments. It was not until the end of the article that it became evident that there were inadequate scientific data to support the effectiveness of the treatments.

Often an article reports on a study of a medical technique or medication, concluding that it has negative aspects, while at the same time warning medical consumers that they should not stop using the treatment because more research needs to be done. When results are inconclusive, medical consumers need to weigh the risks and benefits as they apply specifically to their own conditions and special circumstances.

BUILDING YOUR OWN MEDICAL LIBRARY

Individuals with the inclination and the financial resources may wish to start their own medical reference library. One way to keep up with the latest research and treatment options for a given condition is to subscribe to medical journals in the specialty field that treats the condition. Professional societies for members of the particular medical specialty publish journals that they sell both to libraries and individuals. For example, the American Academy of Ophthalmology publishes the journal, Ophthalmology, and the American Diabetes Association publishes a number of journals, including Diabetes Care. The American Medical Association publishes a number of specialty journals, such as Archives of Internal Medicine, Archives of Ophthalmology, etc. Their journals are listed on their web site (www.ama-assn.org), along with the Tables of Contents from the current issues. If you do not wish to purchase these journals, they are available at medical libraries and some college and university libraries. Although you may not fully understand all that is written in these journals, you may glean enough information to pose additional questions to your physicians. Articles in peer reviewed medical journals have presumably undergone stringent requirements before they are accepted for publication. However, circumstances and funding limitations sometimes preclude using optimal research methods for medical studies. Often editorials accompanying these articles or the articles themselves will point out the limitations of the studies. Readers may also point out limitations and criticisms in subsequent issues of the journal in the letters to the editor section.

Basic reference books are useful for virtually any medical situation. A good basic internal medicine book that covers the organs and systems of the body is essential. You should select a book that is updated on a regular basis in order to include advances in diagnosis and treatment. Two examples of such books are <u>Current Medical Diagnosis and Treatment</u> and <u>Harrison's Principles of Internal Medicine</u>, published by McGraw-Hill Inc. A medical dictionary and a directory of drugs that discusses the use of each drug, side effects, interactions, and contraindications are extremely useful. Books on medical tests describe the procedures, accuracy, discomfort, and risks involved. Two examples are <u>The Patient's Guide to Medical Tests</u>, published by Houghton Mifflin, and <u>The Consumer's Medical Desk Reference</u>, published by the People's Medical Society.

Other good choices for a home medical library include books on topics that cover conditions that affect the family. For example, a woman may wish to purchase books on women's health and gynecology. Individuals with diabetes may wish to build their libraries with the wide variety of books on this topic, including those written for health care providers. By contacting professional societies, it is possible to learn about the vast variety of texts that are available to the professionals who make clinical recommendations. For those unable to purchase these books, medical, university, and public libraries often have these books. Those interested in making purchases may also want to examine them at the library prior to purchase. Check with medical and university libraries prior to making a trip there; although many of these libraries admit the public at no charge, some may charge a fee for the general public to use their collections.

ONLINE RESOURCES

Most libraries now offer access to <u>MEDLINE</u>, a medical database that enables the user to perform searches of the medical literature by topic and author. <u>MEDLINE</u> is also available over the Internet at no charge, directly from the National Library of Medicine, as are several other online databases (see "INTERNET RESOURCES" section below). <u>MEDLINE</u> performs searches of major medical journals and provides citations, abstracts of articles, and in some cases, entire articles. Articles that are not online may be ordered through the organization that provides the service. You may also find the articles at libraries. If your library does not have the articles you want, ask the reference librarians to obtain them from other libraries. Be certain to ask the charge, as it may be less expensive for you to visit the other libraries yourself.

There is anecdotal evidence of individuals who discovered cures for rare and presumably fatal illnesses, cures that their physicians had not been aware of. An extreme example of this phenomenon occurred when the husband of a woman who was dying from a cancer called multiple myeloma discovered in an article on <u>MEDLINE</u> an experimental treatment that had succeeded on mice (Knox: 1995). The author of the article worked at the National Cancer Institute (NCI). The woman's husband convinced the scientist at the NCI to try the experiment on her, requiring an enormous amount of paperwork to obtain government permission. In the end, however, the treatment succeeded, and the woman's cancer regressed. Other less dramatic stories exist about individuals who discovered treatments that cured their disease through <u>MEDLINE</u>.

Many hospitals and medical centers now have their own web sites on the Internet. These sites provide information about the facilities, their departments, and services as well as their medical staff. Some have information especially for medical consumers, such as referrals for physicians, definitions of medical terminology, and links to other medical sites on the Internet.

Other sources available on the Internet include professional organizations of medical specialists. These sites may lead you to a referral for a specialist, list the contents of journals published by the organization, include the full text of articles, or have a database that may be searched by topic. Most professional societies also offer a variety of patient education materials, and some may be downloaded from the Internet. Some sites enable you to ask questions and receive a response from a specialist. Some physicians also have their own web sites where they post articles and respond to questions by e-mail. You may locate these organizations and physicians by going to a search engine such as "altavista.com" and typing in the name of the organization, physician, or the topic.

Internet sites provide access to information from government and service agencies, educational institutions, and commercial organizations. One web site that provides links to information on health is www.yahoo.com. Once at this site, a search by topic results in links to a wealth of information. Another strategy for finding resources related to health is to go to a web site of a service organization that provides links to other health organizations.

Using computers with the Internet and online subscription services, it is possible to communicate with people all over the world. A variety of formats is available to receive and exchange information. When you join a usenet group or a newsgroup, you may read messages and respond to them as well as submit your own information and questions. In order to join a usenet group or a newsgroup, your host computer must provide access. When you subscribe to a usenet group or a newsgroup, you will automatically receive all new messages whenever you log on. If you decide to exchange messages with just one member, you may send mail directly to that individual's e-mail address.

You may also communicate instantly with individuals in similar situations. Chat rooms actually occur in real time; a time is set up when individuals communicate by sending messages and receiving responses immediately. If you participate in a chat room or other online discussion, you should know whether it is moderated and by whom. Moderators guide the participants in areas such as making sure that they stay on the subject and that their language is appropriate. Many of these services are free, with the exception of telephone charges or subscription fees for online services.

Consumers searching for health and medical information online must be aware of the risks as well as the benefits. Quacks and charlatans have the same access to computer technology as do reputable public and private organizations. It is important to check out any information found on the Internet to verify that it is supported by scientific data. The Food and Drug Administration urges consumers to report any suspected fraud related to health and medical issues, such as purported cures and health insurance schemes. E-mail messages may be sent to otcfraud@cder.fda.gov.

Using your common sense is the best way to decide if the information provided is accurate. Was the information provided by an individual or organization credentialed in the health care field? Were references to evaluations of the treatment provided? If so, check them out. Does the language used indicate that the writer is educated and literate? Is the information provided or paid for by an individual or company that is trying to sell a product?

Is the information current? Many web sites post a notice stating that "this page last updated on (date)" or "current as of (date)." How does this site choose the links it provides to other sites? Does the site provide contact information such as mailing address, telephone numbers, or e-mail address so that you can contact the provider?

If you are still uncertain as to the accuracy of the information, look up the topic on MEDLINE. Consult with a physician in the field to see if he or she is familiar with the treatment and any studies that have been conducted to investigate the effectiveness of the treatment and risks or side effects.

TALKING WITH OTHER MEDICAL CONSUMERS

Many medical consumers find it extremely useful to talk with others who have experienced similar health problems in order to learn about the pros and cons of alternative treatments and solutions. Individuals who feel at a loss about locating other individuals with the same problem should start with their own physician. Asking for the names of others who have experienced the same problem will not only provide information from the consumer's perspective, but will also provide information about the quality of care provided by the physician and the facilities involved. If your physician does not have on hand the names of other medical consumers who have volunteered to fill this role, he or she will have to contact the individuals for their permission prior to giving out their names.

Another route to finding individuals with similar conditions is to contact voluntary organizations that are dedicated to helping individuals with the condition. Often, volunteers at the organizations have the conditions themselves, and many of these organizations run their own self-help groups. Examples of these groups are those for men with prostate conditions (the Prostate Cancer Support Network, sponsored by the American Foundation for Urologic Disorders) and for women with breast cancer (Reach to Recovery, sponsored by the American Cancer Society).

Self-help groups offer a number of benefits to participants, including learning to develop coping strategies; acquiring a sense of control over life; combating isolation and alienation; and developing information networks. In addition, members of self-help groups often express a sense of increased self-esteem, because they have offered help to other members of the group.

While exchanging information through chat rooms over the Internet is a recent development in self-help strategies, it is significantly different in character from meeting face-to-face with a group. It provides information and helps to combat social isolation for those in rural areas and those who are unable to leave their homes. It may also serve as a first step in meeting someone with a similar experience who lives in the same geographical area.

The Community Services section of local telephone directories often lists self-help groups under "Health and Human Services" or "Disabilities." The "Social Service Organizations" section of the Yellow Pages is also a good source for locating service agencies and information clearinghouses.

Other sources of self-help groups include directories of local agencies in the public library's reference section; social service or patient education departments of hospitals; and the information and referral service of the local United Way. National self-help clearinghouses, which are centers for information about self-help groups, are listed in the "ORGANI-ZATIONS" section below.

KEEPING A JOURNAL OF YOUR MEDICAL HISTORY

Anyone who experiences medical problems, especially those with unusual and undiagnosed conditions, should keep a journal of symptoms, diagnostic tests, diagnoses, and treatments. If the condition progresses or recurs, even many years later, this journal will help you to recall the prior episodes and how they relate to the progression or recurrence. Write up summaries of any major illnesses, when they occurred, and the course of treatment and its effectiveness. Always take a notebook with you to your doctor's appointments and to the hospital to record the information that you receive. If you have had surgery, list the dates of the operations, reasons for the surgery, and where surgery was performed, as well as problems or symptoms that occurred as a result of the surgery. If you had pre-operative tests, include copies of the results in your records. Obtaining copies of these test results will save you time and money if you consult a different physician for the same medical condition. For this reason, and to be certain that the test results are conveyed to you accurately in a conversation, it is always wise to obtain test results in writing.

Keep a record of medications that you have used for various medical conditions and whether they caused any adverse reactions. Knowing the names of the drugs you are taking is not sufficient; you should inquire into the type of drugs. For example, if you are taking medication for high blood pressure, is the drug a beta-blocker, an ace inhibitor, or a diuretic? Record any drug allergies, such as allergies to penicillin or sulfa drugs. Keep a record of your blood type.

Keeping your medical records organized and up-to-date will help you take charge of your medical care. Whether you use a computer, a notebook, or simple file folders, you should set up a system that gives you easy access to your records. By keeping accurate track of your own medical history, you will avoid the need to wait for a physician's office or a hospital medical records department to send you the results of your prior medical tests, a process which often takes an inordinate amount of time. Tell your physician that you would like copies of all test results sent to you and to note this request in your record. Chances are good that you will have to remind the physician or his or her secretary after each test, despite this notation.

Your medical records will prove useful when seeing a new physician and when filling out insurance or hospital admission forms; they will also provide important information for family members about conditions that may be hereditary. Parents should keep records for their children and make this information available to children when they leave home. A log of physician interactions may also prove valuable if legal action is called for.

Test results, however, are not the only information available in your medical records. Physicians enter notes regarding the physical examinations you received and other observations regarding your health. Frequently, physicians do not tell patients all the details about their conditions and the prognosis for recovery. Specialists who participated in your care usually send a letter to your primary care physician regarding findings of physical examinations, test results, diagnosis, treatment, and prognosis. These letters often contain more detail than the information provided to patients. To obtain the maximum amount of information about your medical history, you should request copies of your medical records to file with test results that you have obtained.

Many states and the federal government have passed laws giving patients the legal right to obtain their medical records. When interviewing a new physician, ask about his or her personal policy regarding medical records. If a physician is reluctant to send your test results to you, discuss the situation. If he or she ultimately refuses to provide you with the records, seek out another physician. You are entitled to receive copies of your hospital records; be persistent and read the material you receive carefully to ensure that the records are complete. Current and former physicians must provide copies of your medical records upon request. Don't rely on the local hospital or doctor's office to keep your records for you. Physicians retire, storage areas are destroyed by floods or fire, or records are simply misfiled. Insist on having copies of your own records.

RE-EVALUATING YOUR MEDICAL CONDITION WITH YOUR PHYSICIAN

Once you have completed your own research on your condition, talked with other medical consumers, and received additional medical opinions, return to your physician and discuss your findings. Some physicians are reluctant to give credence to the fact that many medical consumers are capable of having input into their own medical decisions and may be unwilling to discuss the results of your research. Many physicians feel intimidated by medical consumers who search the medical literature and come into their offices with questions based on what they have read. Some even express the old adage, "A little knowledge is a dangerous thing" and purposely withhold information (Fisher: 1986). If your physician fits this category, tell him or her that you are seeking a new physician, along with the reason for doing so.

In discussing your situation with your physician, take into account your age and your medical history, and ask the physician his or her experience in using various treatment strategies for other patients with similar characteristics. If, in the end, you and your physician disagree on the treatment plan, consult with another physician to determine if your choice for a medical treatment plan is appropriate. However, keep in mind that physicians often express similar opinions based on current medical protocols. In some instances, the protocol is changed in later years, so be wary at the outset and pursue your questioning even in the face of utter confidence on the part of the physicians.

In many instances, medical data are contradictory and confusing regarding the most effective treatment for a condition. An example of a current controversy is the use of hormone replacement therapy in post-menopausal women. While this therapy is often recommended to help prevent heart disease and osteoporosis, some studies have indicated that it increases the risk of breast cancer. Angell (1997), who at the time was the editor of the New England Journal of Medicine, recounted the example of how her journal and the Journal of the American Medical Association published articles that reached opposite conclusions about this topic within a four week period. In such a case, medical consumers must read the studies carefully, take into account the studies' findings related to their own risk factors for the disease involved, and weigh the possible benefits against the possible risks. Such a situation may prove extremely time consuming and may require intensive discussions with physicians who specialize in the area. It is also important to take into account the physicians' own biases before discussing your case. Does the physician always recommend hormone replacement therapy no matter what the woman's individual medical history? In the end, medical consumers must weigh all the factors and take responsibility for their own medical decisions.

CONCLUSION

Armed with the knowledge that it is possible to readily obtain information about medical conditions, diagnostic procedures, and treatments, medical consumers may feel comfortable that they are able to make informed judgments about their own health care. Using online services such as MEDLINE, medical journals, reference books, and textbooks, and talking with others who have gone through similar experiences enables medical consumers to evaluate their own situations and prepare themselves for discussions with their physicians. Additional sources of information to evaluate individual physicians and hospital facilities are discussed in the chapters that follow.

References

Angell, Marcia
1997 "Overdosing on Health Risks" The New York Times Magazine May 4, 44-45
Fisher, Sue
1986 In the Patient's Best Interest: Women and the Politics of Medical Decisions New Brunswick, NJ: Rutgers University Press
Foreman, Judy
1998 "Treatment Options are Growing for Women with Bleeding Disorders" Boston Globe March 23
Knox, Richard A.
1995 "A Case of Cancer Salvation" Boston Globe April 25
Laine, Christine
1994 "A Comparison of Patients' and Physicians' Priorities in Office-Based Health Care" Picker/Commonwealth Report 2:1:(Spring):3
Roter, Debra L. and Judith A. Hall
1989 "Studies of Doctor-Patient Interaction" Annual Review of Public Health 10:163-180
Strull, William M., Bernard Lo, and Gerald Charles
1984 "Do Patients Want to Participate in Medical Decision Making?" JAMA 252:21(December 7):2990-2994

ORGANIZATIONS

Agency for Healthcare Research and Quality (AHRQ)
2101 East Jefferson Street, Suite 501
Rockville, MD 20852
(301) 594-1364   e-mail: info@ahrq.gov   www.ahrq.gov

A federal agency that funds research studies on effectiveness of medical treatments, economic aspects of health care policy, and quality of care. Publishes monthly newsletter, "Research Activities." Free. Newsletter and reports also available on the web site.

American Health Information Management Association (AHIMA)
233 North Michigan Avenue, Suite 2150
Chicago, IL 60601
(312) 233-1100   (FAX) (312) 233-1090
e-mail: info@ahima.org   www.ahima.org

This organization provides a medical records form for adults and children, which may be downloaded from its web site. State chapters of this organization can provide information about state laws regarding patients' rights to their medical records. Addresses of state chapters are available on the web site.

American Self-Help Clearinghouse
100 Hanover Avenue, Suite 202
Cedar Knolls, NJ 07927
(973) 326-6789   FAX (973) 326-9467   www.selfhelpgroups.org

Provides information and contacts for national self-help groups, information on model groups and individuals who are starting new networks, and state or local self-help clearinghouses.

Center for Medical Consumers
130 Macdougal Street
New York, NY 10012
(212) 674-7105   FAX (212) 7100
e-mail: medconsumers@earthlink.net
www.medicalconsumers.org

This organization works at both the state and national level to improve the quality of health care. It works to make the medical system accountable and give the consumer a greater voice in decision-making. The web site has information about medical errors, mammography, drug advertising, and other health topics. Publishes newsletter, "Health Facts," $25.00.

Centers for Disease Control and Prevention (CDC)
1600 Clifton Road, NE
Atlanta, GA 30333
(800) 311-3435   (404) 639-3534   www.cdc.gov

A federal agency that is concerned with a wide range of health issues. Conducts studies and public health programs on major health issues, such as diabetes and AIDS.

Combined Health Information Database (CHID)
Ovid Technologies, Attn: CHID Database
333 7th Avenue
New York, NY 10001
(800) 950-2035   (212) 563-3006   FAX (212) 563-3784
e-mail: chid@aerie.com   chid.nih.gov

A federally sponsored database that includes bibliographic citations and abstracts from journals, reports, medical journals, books, and patient education brochures.

Medical Library Association (MLA)
65 East Wacker Place, Suite 1900
Chicago, IL 60601
(312) 419-9094   FAX (312) 419-8950   e-mail: info@mla.org
www.mlanet.org

The Consumer and Patient Health Information Section of this professional organization for medical librarians evaluates web sites based on credibility, sponsorship/authorship, content, audience, links, and other criteria. A list of health care resources is available on the web site.

National Health Council
1730 M Street, NW, Suite 500
Washington, DC 20036
(800) 684-6814   (202) 785-3910   FAX (202) 785-5923
www.nationalhealthcouncil.org

This association of more than 100 national health organizations includes voluntary health agencies, health-related professional and membership associations, business corporations, and federal agencies. Web site provides information on various conditions.

National Health Information Center (NHIC)
Office of Disease Prevention and Health Promotion
PO Box 1133
Washington, DC 20013-1133
(800) 336-4797   In MD, (301) 565-4167   FAX (301) 984-4256
FAXBACK (301) 468-1204   e-mail: nhicinfo@health.org   nhic-nt.health.org

Maintains a database of health-related organizations and a library. Provides referrals related to health issues for both professionals and consumers. Publications enable individuals to locate information and resources in the federal government. Free publications list. Also available on the web site.

National Institutes of Health (NIH)
9000 Rockville Pike
Building 31, Room 2B03
Bethesda, MD 20892
(301) 496-4143   e-mail: nihinfo@od.nih.gov   www.nih.gov

A federal agency that sponsors research into the causes, prevention, and treatment of disease. Within NIH are a number of institutes that study specific types of diseases. Many of these institutes have publications clearinghouses that provide information to medical consumers as well as professionals. The web site provides links to each of the institutes, and many publications are available on the web site.

National Library of Medicine (NLM)
8600 Rockville Pike
Building 38, Room 2S-10
Bethesda, MD 20894
(888) 346-3656   (301) 594-5983
www.ncbi.nlm.nih.gov/PubMed

Operates PubMed, which provides access to MEDLINE, a computerized database that provides access to articles in major medical journals from around the world. Users may search for a specific health related topic and receive citations and abstracts of articles online. Available directly through NLM, the Internet, and at most medical, public, and university libraries.

National Self-Help Clearinghouse
Graduate School and University Center of the City University of New York
365 5th Avenue, Suite 3300
New York, NY 10016
(212) 817-1822   e-mail: info@selfhelpweb.org   www.selfhelpweb.org

Makes referrals to local self-help groups.

People's Medical Society
462 Walnut Street
Allentown, PA 18102
(800) 624-8773   FAX (610) 770-0607   www.peoplesmed.org

This consumer health advocacy organization publishes books, health bulletins, and fact sheets on many aspects of medical care. Membership, $20.00, includes bimonthly "People's Medical Society Newsletter." The list of publications, "Health Library Catalog," is free.

Quackwatch
PO Box 1747
Allentown, PA 18105
(610) 437-1795   www.quackwatch.com

Established by a physician, this organization is dedicated to combating fraud in health care by investigating questionable claims, answering consumer inquiries, distributing reliable publications, and improving the quality of health information on the Internet. Offers electronic newsletter, "Consumer Health Digest," free.

INTERNET RESOURCES

This section includes resources that are *online resources only.* Organizations that provide services in addition to online resources are listed in the "ORGANIZATIONS" sections, where their Internet addresses are also listed. The number of health related web sites has grown astronomically. By utilizing some of the major sites listed below, you will find links to many other sites.

Center Watch Clinical Trials Listing Service
www.centerwatch.com

Lists clinical trials by general field, such as endocrinology, ophthalmology, etc. Lists new FDA approvals. Links to other health sites on the Internet.

ClinicalTrials.gov
clinicaltrials.gov

This confidential web site has information on more than 4,000 Federal and private medical studies. Lists location of clinical trials, design and purpose, criteria for participation, information about the disease and treatment being studied, and links to personnel who are recruiting participants. Also available at www.nlm.nih.gov.

Consumer.gov
www.consumer.gov

This cooperative project of the Food and Drug Administration, Federal Trade Commission, Consumer Products Safety Commission, National Highway Transportation Safety Administration, and Securities and Exchange Commission offers consumer information on topics such as health and safety, money and credit, children and education, transportation, and food safety. Includes information on FDA warnings and alerts and information for elders.

Dirline
National Library of Medicine (NLM)
8600 Rockville Pike
Building 38, Room 2S-10
Bethesda, MD 20894
(888) 346-3656   (301) 594-5983   dirline.nlm.nih.gov

This database enables the user to search for organizations concerned with specific health conditions.

Health Care Choices
PO Box 21039
Columbia Circle Station, NY 10023
www.healthcarechoices.org

The web site provides physician profiles and information about hospitals, insurance plans, and specific health conditions.

Healthfinder
e-mail: healthfinder@health.org   www.healthfinder.gov

Sponsored by the federal government, this online service provides information about government agencies that are related to health, as well as online publications such as a medical dictionary.

Healthgrades.com
Health Grades
44 Union Boulevard, Suite 600
Lakewood, CO 80228
(303) 716-0041   e-mail: info@.com   www.healthgrades.com

This web site provides consumers assessments of physicians, hospitals, nursing homes, and assisted living facilities. Free

The Healthpages
www.thehealthpages.com

Provides articles on a wide variety of diseases and conditions. Also provides information on physicians and facilities that treat specific disorders in specified metropolitan areas.

HealthWeb
www.healthweb.org

This web site is operated by a consortium of university libraries. The site provides links to a variety of noncommercial health sites that have been evaluated by the librarians.

Librarians' Index to the Internet
lii.org

This searchable, annotated subject directory on Internet resources includes subjects such as disabilities, health, medicine, and seniors.

Mayo Clinic
www.mayohealth.org

This web site provides information about conditions, treatments, and health decisions.

Medem.com
www.medem.com

This web site is a joint venture of national medical societies such as the American Medical Association, American College of Obstetricians and Gynecologists, and the American Academy of Ophthalmology. Offers public information and a Physician Finder.

Medicinenet
www.medicinenet.com

Sponsored by physicians, this web site provides information on diseases, procedures and tests, drugs, a medical dictionary, and links to other health sites.

MEDLINE/PubMed
www.ncbi.nlm.nih.gov/PubMed

This computerized database provides access to articles in major medical journals from around the world. Users may search for a specific health related topic and receive citations and abstracts of articles online. Available directly through NLM, the Internet, and at most medical, public, and university libraries.

Medscape
www.medscape.com

Provides access to full text medical articles. Also has special information for women, a database on AIDS, etc. Sends weekly e-mails about latest medical news. Users may choose to receive e-mails in specific areas of medicine.

National Guideline Clearinghouse
www.guideline.gov

Provides access to hundreds of clinical practice guidelines for common medical conditions and treatments.

National Institutes of Health Information
www.nih.gov/health

Provides a single access point to the National Institutes of Health, including their individual clearinghouses, publications, and the Combined Health Information Database. Provides information on hotlines, MEDLINE, clinical trials and drug information.

Reuters Health Information Services
www.reutershealth.com

Provides current news about health matters.

10 Things to Know About Evaluating Medical Resources on the Web
cancertrials.nci.nih.gov

This list poses questions that consumers should ask when visiting Internet sites that provide medical information. May be downloaded.

WebMDHealth
my.webmd.com

This network provides information about a wide variety health conditions. Includes a special category for conditions affecting women. Operates chat rooms.

PUBLICATIONS

Consumer Reports On Health
Box 56355
Boulder, CO 80322
(800) 333-9784   www.consumerreports.org/service

This monthly publication provides information on topics such as health fraud, health and medical products, prescription and over-the-counter drugs, nutrition, and fitness. $24.00

Columbia University College of Physicans and Surgeons Complete Home Medical Guide
cpmcnet.columbia.edu/texts/guide

An online version of this standard consumer health text.

Consumer's Medical Desk Reference: Information Your Doctor Can't or Won't Tell You
by Charles B. Inlander and the Staff of the People's Medical Society
People's Medical Society
462 Walnut Street
Allentown, PA 18102
(800) 624-8773   FAX (610) 770-0607   www.peoplesmed.org

This book provides information on the medical conditions that affect organs and systems of the body. It discusses criteria for selecting physicians, hospitals, and other medical care settings such as pain clinics, specialized treatment centers, and rehabilitation facilities. Includes chapters on medical tests and risks, family health, medical insurance, consumer protection, and government resources. Members, $14.95; nonmembers, $19.95; plus $4.00 shipping and handling.

Crossing the Quality Chasm: A New Health System for the 21st Century
Committee on Quality of Health Care in America, Institute of Medicine
National Academy Press
2101 Constitution Avenue, NW
Lockbox 285
Washington, DC 20055
(888) 624-8373   (202) 334-3313   FAX (202) 334-2451
e-mail: zjones@nas.edu   www.nap.edu

This book recommends sweeping reforms in the health care delivery system. It documents current practices that negatively affect quality in health care. $44.95 plus $4.50 shipping and handling. Orders placed on the web site receive a discount.

Current Medical Diagnosis and Treatment
by Stephen J. McPhee, Maxine A. Papadakis, and Lawrence M. Tierney (eds.)
McGraw-Hill
7707 Collection Center Drive
Chicago IL 60693
(800) 262-4729   FAX (614) 579-3641
e-mail: customer-service@mcgraw-hill
www.pbg.mcgraw-hill.com/medical/online.htm

Updated annually, this book contains chapters on the organs and systems of the body, the conditions that affect them, and current diagnostic and treatment procedures. $54.95

Harrison's Principles of Internal Medicine
by Eugene Braunwald et al. (eds.)
McGraw-Hill
7707 Collection Center Drive
Chicago IL 60693
(800) 262-4729   FAX (614) 579-3641
e-mail: customer-service@mcgraw-hill
www.pbg.mcgraw-hill.com/medical/online.htm

This book, written by a wide variety of medical specialists and revised periodically, covers virtually every organ and system of the body and the medical problems that affect them. Softcover, $29.95; hardcover, one volume, $125.00; 2 volume set (same content, easier handling, $129.00; CD-ROM $199.00. "Harrison's Online" available with updates for $89.00 annually for single users; www.harrisonsonline.com (800) 773-4607.

Health & Medicine on the Internet 2002
Practice Management Information Group
2001 Butterfield Road, Suite 310
Downers Grove, IL 60515
(800) 633-7467   FAX (800) 633-6556   (323) 954-0224
e-mail: info@medicalbookstore.commedicalbookstore.com

This book describes a variety of Internet sites related to medical conditions, treatments, and chat rooms. $29.95 plus $6.95 shipping and handling

Health-Minder
8000 East Prentice, Suite B-13
Englewood, CO 80111
(303) 220-7449   e-mail: info@Health-Minder.com
www.Health-Minder.com

This software is designed to record personal and family medical history, track medical expenses and insurance, and manage other health information. May be downloaded for a 60 day free trial period. $35.00

JAMA Journal of the American Medical Association
Subscription Services
American Medical Association (AMA)
PO Box 4189
Chicago, IL 60197-9798
(800) 262-2350   (312) 670-7827   FAX (312) 464-5831
e-mail: ama-subs@ama-assn.org   www.ama-assn.org/scipub.htm

A weekly journal that publishes results of current research and other articles of interest to clinicians. Each issue also has a "Patient Page," which discusses a topic related to one of the articles in that issue. $145.00. The table of contents is available free on web site.

Mayo Clinic Health Letter
Mayo Health Information
Subscription Services
PO Box 53889
Boulder, CO 80322-3888
(800) 333-9037   www.mayohealth.org

Monthly newsletter provides information on common health problems, medical techniques, and surgical procedures. $24.00

MemoryMinder Journals
PO Box 23108
Eugene, OR 97402
(800) 888-3392   www.memoryminder.com

The MemoryMinder Personal Health Journal is a spiral-bound health diary that enables users to track daily symptoms, medications, degree of pain or discomfort, dietary intake, and vital signs such as temperature, blood pressure, weight, blood sugar levels, and sleep duration. $12.95 plus $3.50 shipping and handling

Merck Manual of Medical Information - Home Edition
(800) 819-9456   www.merckhomeedition.com

This edition of a classic medical reference provides comprehensive medical information. Available in print, $29.95; CD-ROM, $39.95. The web site offers both a text-based version and an interactive edition, enhanced with photographs, videos, animations, pronunciations, and illustrations.

New England Journal of Medicine
860 Winter Street
Waltham, MA 02451
(800) 843-6356   (781) 893-3800   FAX (781) 893-0413
www.nejm.org

This weekly journal provides articles on recent research and policy issues. The web site provides the table of contents (free) and full text articles may be ordered for $10.00. Back issues may be searched online. Individuals, $135.00; institutions, $399.00.

The Official ABMS Directory of Board Certified Medical Specialties
Reed Elsevier New Providence
PO Box 7247-7781
Philadelphia, PA 19180-7781
(800) 521-8110   www.marquiswhoswho.com

Produced annually by the American Board of Medical Specialties, this directory includes information about physicians' education and training as well as certification by medical specialty boards. $525.00 plus 7 1/2% shipping and handling

Past Imperfect: How Tracing Your Family Medical History Can Save Your Life
by Carol Daus
Santa Monica Press
PO Box 1076
Santa Monica, CA 90406
(800) 784-9553   e-mail: smpress@pacificnet.net
www.santamonicapress.com

This book describes how preparing a genogram, or family health history, can aid families to discover patterns for specific diseases. This information may then be used for genetic counseling or lead to prevention strategies. $12.95 plus $3.00 shipping and handling

PDR Family Guide Encyclopedia of Medical Care
Random House
400 Hahn Road
Westminster, MD 21157
(800) 733-3000   (410) 848-1900   FAX (410) 386-7013
www.randomhouse.com

This book provides information about common medical conditions, treatment, and complications. $23.00 plus $5.50 shipping and handling

PDR Medical Dictionary
Medical Economics Company
PO Box 10689
Des Moines, IA 50336-0689
(800) 678-5689   FAX (515) 284-6714

Contains definitions of medical terms and procedures plus information about generic and brand name pharmaceuticals. $54.95

Personal Health Guide: Put Prevention into Practice
Agency for Healthcare Research and Quality Publications Clearinghouse
PO Box 8547
Silver Spring, MD 20907
(800) 358-9295   (888) 586-6340 (TT)   e-mail: info@ahrq.gov
www.ahrq.gov/ppip/ppadult

This pocket-sized guide enables individuals to record important medical care details such as medication records, immunizations, and preventative tests. Free. Also available on the web site.

The Self-Help Sourcebook Online
American Self-Help Clearinghouse
100 Hanover Avenue, Suite 202
Cedar Knolls, NJ 07927
(973) 326-6789   FAX (973) 326-9467   www.selfhelpgroups.org

This online database provides information on national and model self-help groups, online mutual help groups and networks, and self-help clearinghouses. Includes ideas on starting self-help groups and opportunities to link with others to develop new groups.

Severed Trust: Why American Medicine Hasn't Been Fixed
by George D. Lundberg with James Stacey
Perseus Books Group
5500 Central Avenue
Boulder, CO 80301
(800) 386-5656   e-mail: westvieworders@perseusbooks.com
www.perseusbooks.com

This book views the health care system as one that sacrificed quality for its relationship with the political and commercial systems. It exposes many of the common practices that have failed to serve patients well. $26.00

Stedman's Medical Dictionary
Lipppincott Williams & Wilkins
PO Box 1610
Hagerstown, MD 21741
(800) 638-6423   FAX (303) 449-3356   www.lww.com

This reference book defines more than 100,000 medical words and terms. $49.95 plus $5.50 shipping and handling. CD-ROM, $79.95 plus $9.00 shipping and handling

Taber's Cyclopedic Medical Dictionary
F. A. Davis
1915 Arch Street
Philadelphia, PA 19103
(800) 323-3555   FAX (215) 440-3016
e-mail: orders@fadavis.com   www.fadavis.com

A medical dictionary with a variety of appendices, including medical emergencies, medical abbreviations, and anatomy. $32.95; with thumbed index, $35.95; multimedia CD-ROM which runs on Windows or Macintosh, $49.95.

The Wellness Letter
University of California at Berkeley
Subscription Department
PO Box 420148
Palm Coast, FL 32142
(386) 447-6328   www.berkeleywellness.com

This monthly newsletter stresses physical, mental, and emotional well-being. $28.00

Chapter 2

LOCATING APPROPRIATE HEALTH CARE

In order to obtain quality health care, it is important to find physicians who understand not only your disease or condition, but also your need for information and to participate in the decision-making process. While such a quest will take more time than simply selecting a physician from a telephone listing, a referral service, or a friend or relative's suggestion, in the end, you are more likely to be satisfied with your choice. Variables such as age, gender, education, location, and specialty may all play a part in your choice of a physician. In addition, it is crucial that you have the type of health insurance plan that permits you to select a compatible physician. Strategies for selecting both physicians and health care plans are discussed below.

FINDING A COMPATIBLE PHYSICIAN

Obtaining information about a specific medical condition often takes place in times of stress. After all, no one can predict when a medical problem may strike. One way of being prepared is to have a relationship with a primary care physician that you trust. This physician should respect your right to obtain information about your condition and treatment options. When the primary care physician is unable to treat the condition, he or she may help you nonetheless by referring you to a specialist who works in the field.

Some individuals feel more comfortable with the services of a physician who is of the same gender they are. As more women become physicians, more information becomes available about differences between male and female practice styles. One study found that female physicians are significantly more likely to conduct longer visits with patients than male physicians. The same study found that female physicians are more likely to spend time building "partnerships" with patients, asking questions, and providing information (Roter et al.: 1991). Another study found that longer visits are more likely to increase patient participation in decision-making and that male patients seeing male physicians have less participatory visits than male patients seeing female physicians or female patients seeing physicians of either gender (Kaplan et al.: 1995).

Selecting a physician who is both competent and compatible with your personal needs may be the most difficult step in obtaining quality care. Obtaining information about the physician, including his or her credentials and experience, is the first step in the process. Most guide books recommend that patients check the physician's credentials, including medical training, medical specialty, and board certification. This information is necessary but far from complete. Although there have been some noted exceptions of individuals who have practiced "medicine" without proper training or credentials, virtually all practicing physicians have had medical training.

The physician's level of performance since his or her training and certification, which involves passing an examination given by the medical specialty board, may have changed. Many states require that physicians attend continuing medical education courses in order to have their licenses renewed, and some specialty boards require periodic re-certification (emergency medicine, family practice, general surgery, obstetrics/gynecology, orthopedics, thoracic surgery, and urology [Bradley: 1994]), but these requirements are far from universal. Furthermore, it is not illegal for a physician to state that he or she is a specialist without having had special training or certification in that area.

If you live in an area that has one or more medical schools, you may want to begin your search by checking out the specialists and subspecialists within the departments relevant to your needs. Another method is to carry out a MEDLINE search (see Chapter 1, "INTERNET RESOURCES" section) search by subject to determine if any physicians in your area have written articles on your condition.

OBTAINING INFORMATION ABOUT PHYSICIANS

Getting information about the physician and his or her practice prior to making an appointment will save time and frustration later on. It is important to inquire whether the physician has had any malpractice cases where the finding went against him or her, although out of court settlements and jury decisions may not be a true indicator of the physician's negligence. However, when physicians have a pattern of malpractice suits against them, it is wise to question their competence. The state medical licensing board should have information about physicians who have had malpractice cases with an insurance company paying out for the claim, whether the board itself or any hospital has taken disciplinary actions against the physicians, or whether individuals have filed complaints. Searching court records where the physician has practiced is another method of determining if the physician has been involved in malpractice suits, although this method may be quite cumbersome. A competent physician should not hesitate to answer your questions about malpractice suits and explain the situation if he or she has had any suits decided against him or her.

The state of Massachusetts Board of Registration in Medicine was the first state agency to make public information about physicians' training, specialties, certifications, publications, disciplinary actions taken by a hospital, and payments made on malpractice cases. This information is available both by telephone request and over the Internet. Other states also provide basic information about physicians over the Internet (www.docboard.org), although they do not provide information about publications, malpractice cases, or disciplinary actions taken by hospitals or licensing boards. The federal government maintains the National Practitioner Data Bank which contains information about physicians who have lost their license to practice in one state or who have been disciplined by a hospital or health maintenance organization (HMO) in order to prevent them from obtaining a license in another state. Unfortunately, this information is not available to the general public. The law does require, however, that hospitals and HMOs check this database before offering clinical privileges to a physician.

Physicians who have had their licenses revoked in one state may practice legally in another state. Despite the fact that state licensing boards report the revocation of licenses to the Federation of State Medical Boards, some physicians hold licenses to practice in more than one state and therefore may set up practice in another state without re-applying for a license. If their license has been revoked in one state, the second state may not learn about the revoked license.

Information about physicians is also available from a variety of other sources, such as the <u>Directory of Physicians in the United States</u>, available in the reference section of many public and medical libraries, and membership directories of professional societies of physicians.

Obtaining this basic information is only the first step in selecting a competent, compatible physician. Many people consult with friends and relatives to locate a new physician. Their advice is only valuable if they are looking for the same characteristics in a physician that you are. Your elderly aunt may hold the philosophy that "doctors know best," and not require any information to justify the physician's advice. You, on the other hand, may want medical references on the pros and cons of the recommended treatment to assure yourself that it is really the best one for you. You may want a physician whose practice is structured to maximize patient input into decision-making regarding medical treatment, whereas some of your friends may feel that they are too busy to become deeply involved in the decision-making process. Therefore, their recommendations for a physician would not be of value to you. On the other hand, you may have relatives, friends, or acquaintances who have similar values and interests regarding medical care; the advice of these individuals would prove more valuable.

Obtaining Information from the Physician's Office

Judging a physician's technical competence and his or her "bedside manner" is often difficult for the medical consumer. Most individuals judge physicians on the personal attributes the physician exhibits toward them (DiMatteo et al.: 1979). When making an appointment for a first visit with a physician, ask the receptionist about the physician's practices. For example:

> • Does the physician have a hospital affiliation and if so, which hospital?
> • In a group practice, do patients always see the same physician, or do they see whoever is available?
> • Does the physician use "physician extenders" (nurse practitioners and physician assistants), and if so, what roles do they play in the exam?
> • Who covers when the physician is unavailable?
> • Does the physician see patients immediately when an urgent medical situation occurs?
> • What types of health insurance plans does the physician accept?
> • Does the physician have special hours when phone calls are taken from patients? Does the physician answer phone calls and provide test results himself or herself, or does an assistant do this? Nurses and other assistants may be capable of answering some rudimentary questions, but questions specific to a medical condition and its treatment should be answered personally by the physician.
> • Individuals who have physical disabilities should inquire about accessibility. For suggested questions, see Chapter 9.

This initial encounter with the receptionist may provide some preliminary information about the physician's practices. A willingness to answer your questions over the phone indicates that the practice is likely to provide patients with the information they need. A receptionist who does not have the time to answer these questions or seems brusque probably reflects a practice that is overextended and understaffed.

Obtaining Information during Your Meeting with the Physician

You should have the opportunity to meet with the physician while you are fully clothed, prior to the examination (Bontke: 1994). You also should have the right to bring along a person that you trust -- a spouse, a partner, or a good friend -- to act as your advocate. This is especially helpful during first visits or when you have a serious health condition. Anxieties caused by a first meeting or by a serious health problem may cause medical consumers to fail to hear all that the physician says, while the advocate may be capable of remembering.

You (and your advocate) should meet privately with the physician. You should repeat the questions you asked over the phone. It is helpful to bring along a list of written questions. Asking the physician whether he or she attends professional meetings, reads medical journals, or takes continuing medical education courses provides information about his or her interest in staying up-to-date on current medical treatments. In addition, questions regarding specific treatment philosophies should be discussed, especially if you have a medical condition that needs treatment. Judging the physician's personal attributes and technical competence may rely upon several criteria. Is the physician willing to answer your questions without appearing threatened or telling you that you do not need the information? A physician who is secure in his or her competence should not feel threatened by a patient's questions. Competent physicians should respond fully to a patient's questions, providing sources of medical literature, and in some circumstances, providing the names of other patients who have undergone the same treatment or procedure.

In some instances, you may find that the physician has not mentioned a specific treatment that you read about in your review of the medical literature. In this instance, you should raise the issue of this treatment and ask the physician whether or not it would be appropriate in your case. You may find that the physician did not mention the treatment because a certain aspect of your condition is not amenable with the treatment. Alternatively, you may find that the physician is not familiar with the treatment or has a bias against it. Studies have found that treatments vary not only by gender of physician and patients, but also by physician specialty and geographic region. For example, a study found that neurologists and internists were more likely to prescribe aspirin or other platelet antiagents as a prevention for stroke than surgeons were (Goldstein et al.: 1996).

Nor should the physician feel threatened by the request for a second opinion. A second opinion may simply confirm the original diagnosis, but it may provide you with treatment alternatives. If you decide to see a specialist or seek a second opinion, you should tell your current physician of your decision and ask for copies of your medical records to take with you, (if you don't have them already). Be sure to check with your health care plan to verify that a second opinion is covered. In order to get an independent second opinion, go to a physician who is in another practice and who is affiliated with a different hospital than the original physician. Many voluntary organizations that deal with the specific condition or primary care physicians are able to provide the names of specialists in the field. Use the same criteria for selecting this physician as you did when you selected the first physician.

Try to overcome your anxieties about broaching these topics by remembering that it is your body that you are trying to protect. By appearing articulate and informed, you will impress the physician with your knowledge and interest in being a joint decision-maker in your own health care. Start by coming prepared to provide a succinct medical history and with copies of any relevant medical records in your possession. Bring articles related to your condition to discuss with the physician.

Evaluating Your Encounter with the Physician

You should determine if the physician has a conservative approach (generally, he or she waits and monitors the condition before initiating treatment) or an aggressive approach (usually intervenes early and intensively, ordering tests and recommending surgery) (Stutz et al.: 1990). Discussing the physician's recommended treatment for a specific condition is the best way to determine the physician's orientation. The physician's communication style is another factor to consider. A study reported that a physician's negative communication behaviors increases the risk of malpractice suits when patients perceive that the physician is at fault or uncertain about the reason for bad outcomes (Lester and Smith: 1993).

In an attempt to evaluate your interactions with the physician, you may wish to ask yourself the following about your experience:

- Did I get an appointment within a reasonable period of time?
- Did I get to see the physician promptly?
- Was the initial interview conducted before I was asked to disrobe?
- Did the physician conduct the examination, or did a nurse practitioner or physician assistant conduct the examination?
- Did the physician treat me respectfully? Did he or she address me by my first name but introduce himself or herself as "Dr.?"
- Did the physician encourage me to ask questions? Did he or she answer them to my satisfaction? Or did the physician feel threatened by my questions and say that I did not need the information I requested? Did he or she seem distracted and not able to concentrate on my concerns?
- Did the exam seem thorough? As thorough as those I've had with other physicians?
- Did the physician skip procedures that some people find embarrassing, such as a rectal exam?
- Did the physician seem rushed during the appointment? Did he or she interrupt when I was speaking? Did he or she answer telephone calls during the appointment?
- Did the physician describe the diagnosis in clear terms and make certain that I understood?

• Did the physician pay adequate attention to my emotional response to the diagnosis of a serious condition?

• Did the physician present alternative treatment options and then seek out my opinion?

• Did the physician provide thorough instructions for using a prescription drug, including information about side effects and interactions with other drugs or food and alcohol?

• Does the physician's approach to medical treatment seem compatible with my own, i.e., does he or she take a wait-and-see approach or a more aggressive approach?

• Did the physician phone me promptly with the results of lab tests? Did he or she send me copies of my test results when I requested them? Did he or she provide a written interpretation of the results with suggestions for treatment?

• How did the physician respond to my request to seek a second opinion? If the response was positive, were any recommendations made?

If the answers to these questions and others are satisfactory to you, the physician you have seen apparently meets your needs. When you make the decision to continue seeing a particular physician, you should have your records transferred to the new physician. If you have copies of all your previous test results, make copies for the new physician.

If the answers to the above questions are not satisfactory to you, you may wish to reconsider whether this physician is right for you. Expressing your dissatisfaction with the physician may improve the situation, but if you still are not satisfied that the situation will improve, you should seek out a different physician. It is wise to begin this process when you are healthy, if possible; looking for a new physician during a health crisis creates a very stressful situation. While focusing on your immediate health problem, you may find it very difficult to apply the criteria you would under normal conditions.

You should continuously evaluate your physician as your relationship goes on. Physicians and their practice styles may change over time. A physician who seemed compassionate and interested in his or her patients when first starting in practice may have less time to spend with patients as the practice grows. Such changes for the worse may prove not only extremely frustrating, but also may result in a poor quality of care. Furthermore, physicians who are overworked in their office practices have less time to keep abreast of recent developments in their fields by reading medical journals and attending professional meetings. When these characteristics appear in your physician's practice, it is time to seek out a different physician. You should ask yourself the same questions about a physician with whom you have had an ongoing relationship as you would for a new physician.

In some instances, you may conduct a review of the medical literature on a specific condition and find that your physician is not familiar with the literature. In cases where you are otherwise satisfied with the physician, you may wish to discuss your findings and ask the physician if he or she will undertake a literature review. If this is your first visit with the physician, or if treatment requires surgery, it may be wise to find another physician who is familiar with the literature and has experience with the current treatment options.

A physician who admits that he or she is unfamiliar with your symptoms is not necessarily a bad doctor; rather, the physician is admitting his or her limitations. In an era of highly specialized medicine, such limitations are not a sign of incompetence. In such an instance, the physician should refer you to a competent specialist who is qualified to deal with the situation. If the situation is urgent, a referral to a specialist should be obtained at once. Physicians may make referrals to specialists in good faith, thinking that their colleagues have good communication skills and competencies that are compatible with your needs. If this turns out not to be the case, contact your primary care physician, explain the situation, and ask for another referral. If the physician does not know another specialist or declines to make another referral, use the methods described above to locate a specialist on your own, bringing with you your medical history that is relevant to the current problem.

It is not unusual for a number of specialists to be involved in diagnosing and treating a patient. It is not unusual for the opinions of these practitioners to vary, providing conflicting explanations and recommended treatments and causing confusion for the patient. In this situation, you should request that the physicians meet to discuss your case, with you and the physician you consider to be the most knowledgeable and informed about your situation as the case managers. If it is not possible to have an actual face-to-face meeting with all of the physicians, a conference call may be arranged. Or the physician of your choice may request written opinions from the various consulting specialists and then meet with you to discuss the pros and cons of each recommendation.

WHEN THE PHYSICIAN SAYS YOUR SYMPTOMS ARE PSYCHOSOMATIC

It is not uncommon for physicians to attribute ailments that they do not understand to psychological causes. Physicians are especially likely to take this approach when the patient is a woman. However, virtually all patients are vulnerable to this diagnosis, which may sometimes turn out to be dangerous or deadly. When an individual has a rare condition that the physician is unable to diagnose, it is commonplace for the physician to attribute the symptoms to psychosomatic factors.

Edward Rosenbaum (1988), a prominent physician himself, wrote about his experience obtaining the proper diagnosis of a tumor in his throat. Rosenbaum was having difficulty speaking and sought medical advice. Two physicians examined him, a biopsy performed by the pathology laboratory yielded negative results, and he was told that his condition was psychological. His unsatisfactory interactions with physicians continued for six months before he was diagnosed with cancer. Even though he was a physician, he felt intimidated to ask the questions he wanted the physicians to answer.

When a physician tells you that there is nothing wrong, asks if you are under "stress," and implies or states that your condition is psychological, and you believe otherwise, seek another opinion. Should other physicians repeat the same diagnosis, seek out help from a voluntary organization that provides patient advocacy services or self-help groups where others with similar conditions can tell you how they obtained proper health care. Finding a physician who will listen to your complaints and take them seriously may take a lot of work and perseverance. However, in the long run, you may be saving your health and your life.

WHEN THE PHYSICIAN SAYS NOTHING MORE CAN BE DONE

It is not at all unusual for physicians to tell patients that "There is nothing more that can be done." While it may be true that medical and surgical interventions have been exhausted, physicians have a responsibility to help the patients learn to cope with the condition and in the case of disabling conditions, to remain as independent as possible.

DeWitt Stetten, a physician himself, described his experiences with medical professionals when he was diagnosed with age-related macular degeneration, a condition that results in the loss of central vision:

> Through all these years and despite many contacts with skilled and experienced professionals, no ophthalmologist has at any time suggested any device that might be of assistance to me. No ophthalmologist has mentioned any of the many ways in which I could stem the deterioration of my life. (1981:458)

In making referrals for rehabilitation services, physicians have a unique opportunity to empower their patients to adjust to life with a disability or chronic condition.

If you develop a disabling or chronic condition, you can advocate for yourself by asking questions such as:

- What organizations exist that help people with my condition?
- Do you have any literature that discusses how others cope with this condition?
- Is there a support group that I can join? What about support for my family?

A competent, compatible physician will not hesitate to answer these questions or to refer you to someone who can help you obtain this information. Physicians should provide patients with educational literature about their condition and services available to help them, including support groups (see Chapter 9, "People with Chronic Illnesses and Disabilities and the Health Care System").

ALTERNATIVE MEDICINE

When physicians do not offer a cure for a given condition, some consumers seek other sources of help, often in the form of alternative medicine. The term alternative medicine is used to describe treatment methods that are not part of mainstream medical practice. Because alternative medical techniques have often not been tested for effectiveness or safety, they are unlikely to be found in hospitals and are not generally covered by health insurance. A study showed that one in three patients used alternative therapies; it also found that nearly three-quarters of these patients did not tell their physicians they were using unconventional treatments concurrently (Eisenberg: 1993).

The National Institutes of Health has established the National Center for Complementary and Alternative Medicine (NCCAM) (see "ORGANIZATIONS" section below). Research projects sponsored by NCCAM are currently investigating treatments such as biofeedback, acupuncture, hypnosis, imagery, and electrical current therapy in clinical trials (Stehlin: 1996). As with any therapy, use caution when considering alternative medical treatment. Gather as much information as possible about the treatment, such as risks, benefits, and costs, and ask about the credentials of the individual who will provide the treatment. Conduct a MEDLINE search to determine if any scientific studies testing the effectiveness of the treatment have been reported. Talk to others who have used the treatment about their experiences in the short and long run. Discuss the treatment with your primary care physician, since a new treatment might affect or interfere with your conventional medical treatments.

REFUSING MEDICAL TREATMENT
(Also see Chapter 5, "ADVANCE DIRECTIVES" section)

Patients have the right to refuse medical treatment. From the refusal of a simple diagnostic procedure such as measuring body temperature to major surgery that may save a life, a patient may not be forced to "comply" with medical recommendations. In the case of minors, however, where parents or guardians refuse to treat serious medical conditions, advocates for children have stepped in and obtained court orders to initiate treatment.

Many medical consumers view physicians' recommendations for treatment as too aggressive and dangerous. For example, a woman who had had diabetes for 40 years stepped on a staple and developed an infection in her foot. Several physicians told her that her foot would have to be amputated. She rejected their advice and visited a podiatrist, who prescribed a lengthy course of antibiotic treatment and debridement of her infection three times weekly. Two years after the initial incident, she still had her foot, in spite of her physicians' advice (Taliaferro: 1997).

While not all cases of rejecting physicians' advice turn out so well, recommended treatments vary by geographic area and physician specialty, suggesting that not all medical treatment is supported by scientific evidence that it is the best course. After obtaining all the information you can about your condition and possible treatments, you are the one who is the final judge of what should be done.

WHEN SOMETHING GOES WRONG

Even when medical consumers follow the necessary steps to try to ensure that they will receive the best possible treatment, medical practitioners may still make mistakes, some of them deadly. For example, Sandy Gilbert and her husband Elliot, both college professors, consulted more than a half dozen physicians and researched Elliot's condition, prior to his surgery for prostate cancer:

But as alert consumers of medical care, we'd also been determined to review and research all Elliot's options ourselves. We called an old friend, a pathologist at the National Institutes of Health (NIH) in Washington, and asked his advice about doctors and treatments. . . we were assimilated into an informal prostate cancer network, local survivors of the disease who were glad to talk in person or on the phone about the choices they'd made. . .we did an on-line computer search of the medical literature ourselves. . . in our determination to make the right decision about the management of my husband's case. (Gilbert: 1995, pp. 28-29)

Despite these efforts to seek the best medical care, Elliot Gilbert died from post-surgical complications, apparently the result of poorly performed surgery. In the end, it is not possible to monitor procedures in the operating room or the recovery room. For this reason, it is especially important to have confidence that both the surgeon and the facility are competent and properly equipped to handle the procedure (see Chapter 4, "Protecting Yourself in the Hospital").

It is often difficult to determine whether to sue a physician and a health care facility in the event of unanticipated negative outcomes. The majority of medical malpractice suits are found in favor of the physicians and the facilities. Nonetheless, if you feel that a medical procedure or treatment has caused you harm due to negligence on the part of the physician or the facility or that a loved one's death was due to medical error or negligence, speak to an attorney who specializes in this area. Possible options prior to bringing suit include out of court settlement and arbitration. Even when a suit is filed, most cases are settled before they go to trial. Most attorneys accept medical malpractice cases on a contingency basis, that is, they are paid only if they win the case. However, other expenses, such as paying expert witnesses and obtaining medical records must be paid by the plaintiff, even if the plaintiff loses the case.

WHAT TO DO IF THE PHYSICIAN IS IMPAIRED

Physicians have a high rate of drug addiction, in part due to their easy access to controlled substances. The rate of alcoholism is two times greater than drug addiction or mental illness among physicians (Bradley: 1994). In order to satisfy their own addiction, impaired physicians sometimes steal drugs that were meant for their patients. Using drugs that were meant for patients and then performing operations under the influence of drugs present a danger for patients. A code of silence often protects impaired physicians. Physicians who are impaired by virtue of alcoholism, drug addiction, or a disease that affects their mental functioning should be reported to their supervisors and to the state medical licensing board. The American Medical Association Code of Ethics requires physicians who are aware of a colleague's impairment to take action, otherwise he or she may be held liable for any injury that occurs to a patient as a result of the physician's impairment (Hughes: 1995). Instead of disciplining impaired physicians, many state medical licensing boards now conduct treatment programs to help impaired physicians overcome their addictions (Voelker: 1994). If you are uncertain whether a physician is impaired, discuss your suspicions with a friend who also sees the same physician or another physician whom you trust.

CHOOSING A HEALTH CARE PLAN

Choosing a health care provider is often limited by the requirements of a particular health care plan. Traditionally, health care in the United States has been provided on a fee-for-service basis, where the provider billed either the insurance company or the patient for each service rendered. While many Americans still use this type of health care, the number of individuals who use "managed care" plans is growing rapidly. "Managed care" plans were developed in an attempt to control health care costs. "Managed care" is a term that is used to cover a variety of health care plans where the plan's administrators control the way health care is delivered. In health maintenance organizations (HMOs), preventative health is stressed, and usually the care is provided by professionals who are salaried members of the staff.

Some of these plans allow patients to select a primary care physician that they see whenever they have a health concern. Other plans do not permit patients to select physicians; rather, patients see whatever physician is available when they require medical attention. In order to see a specialist, the primary care physician must make a referral. A number of large HMOs have eased this requirement, permitting patients to see specialists at any time, without a referral. The reason for easing this requirement is that competing plans that allow patients to decide on their own to go to a specialist have been luring patients away from the plans that require "gatekeepers" for a referral to a specialist. It is always wise to consider if the physician is prescribing a procedure in order to increase his or her income. Obtaining a second opinion from a physician at another facility should help you determine the answer to this question. On occasions when patients require the services of a specialist that is not a member of the staff, the plan determines which specialist will provide the care.

Preferred provider organizations (PPOs) enable members to select from a larger pool of physicians, but the services of those who are deemed "preferred" cost the members far less. These physicians still maintain private practices but have developed financial arrangements with the insurer. If you are interested in using the services of a particular physician or physicians, check the list of preferred providers to make sure that physician is on the list. If you are looking for a new primary care physician or specialist, call the offices of some of the physicians listed to ensure that they are still part of the PPO network and that they are accepting new patients prior to enrolling in the plan.

The demands of managed care may require that providers spend less time with patients. In fact, some managed care plans have developed target goals for the amount of time physicians spend with patients, thereby limiting the time spent with any individual patient (Knox: 1996). A past president of the Massachusetts Medical Society was quoted as follows:

> With fee-for-service, physicians are paid for what they do. Under
> some managed care plans, they are paid for what they don't do.
> (Pham: 1996)

This quote clearly points to inadequacies in both types of systems. In fee-for-service systems, physicians often order tests to increase the revenue for their institution. Providers may be encouraged to prescribe more services than necessary when the institution receives payment on a fee-for-service arrangement. According to the federal government, half of all Americans now receive their health care through HMOs (Agency for Health Care Policy and Research: 1997). In managed care, where the health plan receives the same compensation per patient no matter how many procedures are performed, physicians are rewarded for not ordering tests. In order to optimize profits, physicians often spend less time with patients than what is optimal to provide quality care. They may be rewarded for providing fewer costly services when the insurance pays a flat fee per patient no matter the amount of services provided. In either case, it is not the patient's health that drives the physician's decisions.

A study of Medicare recipients who had experienced a stroke compared the care provided by HMOs and that provided by fee-for-service plans. The study found that patients whose health care was provided by HMOs were less likely to be discharged from the hospital and sent to rehabilitation centers than patients whose health care was provided by fee-for-service plans. This finding suggests that HMOs may skimp on the care they provide to these patients, possibly denying them rehabilitative services. It should be noted that the study did not evaluate the type of treatment received or the patients' level of functioning (Retchin et al.: 1997).

Health care professionals themselves are beginning to question the efficacy of the managed care system. In the summer of 1997, members of the faculty of the Harvard Medical School held a press conference where they parodied the failings of managed care (American Society on Aging: 1997). Among their criticisms of HMOs were their failure to provide adequate benefits and their lack of attention to problems of elderly patients. Thousands of physicians and nurses in Massachusetts staged a protest against for-profit health care providers, urging their colleagues not to treat patients as profit centers (Kong: 1997). In addition, physicians and dentists in many states have begun to unionize, as their ability to make independent medical decisions regarding their patients has been largely curtailed by insurance companies and managed care organizations (Tye: 1997). They believe that they may regain some of the independence that they have lost by negotiating collectively with insurers. Some critics have asserted that managed care plans work best for healthy, young individuals.

Most large employers offer a variety of health care plans, so employees may select the one that best fits their needs and budgets. Before signing up for a plan, you should get literature from each plan you are considering and compare them carefully. Consider the following when making a decision:

> • How does the plan select physicians? Are they all board certified
> in their fields?
> • How are physicians compensated? Is there an incentive system
> for physicians to keep medical costs down?
> • Do I get to select my own primary care physician, or must I see
> the physician who happens to be available at the time of my
> appointment?
> • How are out-of-state and emergency situations handled?

• How does the cost of the plan compare with fee-for-service plans?
• How does the plan deal with conditions when the appropriate type
of specialist is not affiliated with the plan?
• Is there a formal process for appealing medical decisions?

There is an abundance of literature discussing the different types of managed care plans (see "PUBLICATIONS" section below), the advantages and disadvantages of each type, along with comparisons of managed care plans with fee-for-service plans. After reviewing the literature, make a list of questions, determine if the answers are provided in brochures from the plan itself, determine if state law has specific requirements for managed care plans, and then present your remaining questions to officials of the plans you are considering. Selecting a health care plan based solely on the relative cost is not a wise idea. The benefits provided are usually dependent upon the cost of the plan. Although you may feel that you are fit and healthy, a major purpose of health insurance is to cover the costs of unexpected medical care. Saving money at the outset in lower premiums may result in paying more when the need for care occurs.

At the time this book went to press Congress and the President were debating provisions of "The Patients' Bill of Rights." Under this proposed legislation, patients would have the right to sue HMOs. Under debate were issues such as whether a cap should be imposed on the awards patients could receive as a result of litigation and, if so, how much it would be and whether the litigation should take place in state or federal courts.

References

Agency for Health Care Policy and Research
1997 "Primary Care Research" Research Activities January
American Society on Aging
1997 "Harvard Docs Announce 'HMO Black'" Aging Today September/October p. 8
Bontke, Catherine
1994 "Patient Rights and Your Physician" Abled IV:3(Fall):12-15
Bradley, Edward L.
1994 Patient's Guide to Surgery Philadelphia, PA: University of Pennsylvania Press
DiMatteo, M. Robin, Louise M. Prince, and Angelo Taranta
1979 "Patients' Perceptions of Physicians' Behavior: Determinants of Patient Commitment
    to the Therapeutic Relationships" Journal of Community Health 4:4(Summer):280-290
Eisenberg, D.M. et al.
1993 "Unconventional Medicine in the United States" New England Journal of Medicine
    328:4(January 28):246-52
Gilbert, Sandra
1995 Wrongful Death: A Medical Tragedy New York, NY: W. W. Norton & Company
Goldstein, Larry et al.
1996 "U.S. National Survey of Physicians' Practices for the Secondary and Tertiary
    Prevention of Ischemic Stroke" Stroke 27:9:473-1478

Hughes, Patrick H. et al.

1995 "What To Do When a Colleague Is Impaired" <u>Patient Care</u> 29:12(July 15):117-125

Kaplan, S.H. et al.

1995 "Patient and Visit Characteristics Related to Physicians: Participatory Decision-Making Style: Results from the Medical Outcomes Study" <u>Medical Care</u> 33:12(December): 1176-1197

Knox, Richard A.

1996 "The Rush is on - in Doctors' Offices" <u>Boston Globe</u> March 2

Kong, Dolores

1997 "Doctors, Nurses Condemn For-Profit Care" <u>Boston Globe</u> December 3

Lester, Gregory W. and Susan G. Smith

1993 "Listening and Talking to Patients: A Remedy for Malpractice Suits" <u>Western Journal of Medicine</u> 158:268-272

Pham, Alex

1996 "Fee Systems May Affect Doctor Care" <u>Boston Globe</u> August 11

Retchin, Sheldon M. et al.

1997 "Outcomes of Stroke Patients in Medicare Fee for Service and Managed Care" <u>JAMA</u> 278:2:(July 9):119-124

Rosenbaum, Edward E.

1988 <u>A Taste of My Own Medicine: When the Doctor is the Patient</u> New York, NY: Random House

Roter, D., M. Lipkin Jr. and A. Korsgaard

1991 "Sex Differences in Patients' and Physicians' Communication during Primary Care Medical Visits" <u>Medical Care</u> 29:11(November):1083-1093

Stehlin, Isadora B.

1995 "An FDA Guide to Choosing Medical Treatments" <u>FDA Consumer</u> Rockville, MD: U.S. Food and Drug Administration

Stetten, DeWitt

1981 "Coping with Blindness" <u>New England Journal of Medicine</u> 305:8(August 20):458-460

Stutz, David R., Bernard Feder, and the Editors of Consumer Reports

1990 <u>The Savvy Patient: How to Be an Active Participant in Your Medical Care</u> Mt. Vernon, NY: Consumers Union

Taliaferro, Brenda

1997 "A Second Opinion" <u>Voice of the Diabetic</u> 12:3(Summer):4

Tye, Larry

1997 "MDs Examine Benefits of Unionizing" <u>Boston Globe</u> November 14

Voelker, Rebecca

1994 "Finding Effective Treatment for Impaired Physicians" <u>JAMA</u> 272:16(October 26):1238

ORGANIZATIONS

American Academy of Family Physicians (AAFP)
11400 Tomahawk Creek Parkway
Leawood, KS 66211-2672
(913) 906-6000   e-mail: fp@aafp.org   www.aafp.org
familydoctor.org

This professional membership organization represents physicians who specialize in family practice. Publishes clinical journal, "American Family Physician," 24 times a year; physicians, $83.00; health care professionals, $52.00; institutions, $99.00. The web site, familydoctor.org, provides information about common medical concerns, drugs, herbs and alternative treatments, and self-care flowcharts.

American Board of Medical Specialties (ABMS)
1007 Church Street, Suite 404
Evanston, IL 60201
(866) 275-2267   (847) 491-9091   FAX (847) 328-3596
www.abms.org

This organization will tell consumers if a particular physician is board certified and provide a list of certified specialists by field and geographic region. Services also available at the web site.

American Medical Association (AMA)
515 North State Street
Chicago, IL 60610
(312) 464-5000   www.ama-assn.org

The major professional organization representing physicians in the U.S., the AMA publishes numerous professional journals, including JAMA (Journal of the American Medical Association) and journals for medical specialties. The tables of contents for these journals are available on the AMA's web site. Also available online is "AMA Physician Select," which enables users to locate physicians by specialty and geographic area as well as to check individual physician's credentials.

Association of State Medical Board Executive Directors
www.docboard.org

A growing number of states are joining this online database that lists the training, credentials, board certification, length of time in practice, and licenses of physicians in their state. Some states include information about malpractice suits against the physicians.

Best Doctors in America
1359 Silver Bluff Road, Suite F6
Aiken, SC 29803
(800) 675-1199   FAX (803) 648-7076
e-mail: info@bestdoctors.com   www.bestdoctors.com

A service that locates doctors who are highly rated by their peers to treat the specific conditions described by callers. Fees vary.

Centers for Medicare and Medicaid Services (CMS)
formerly Health Care Financing Administration (HCFA)
7500 Security Boulevard
Baltimore, MD 21244
(800) 633-4227   (410) 786-3000   www.ssa.gov
www.medicare.gov

CMS is the federal agency that administers Medicare and Medicaid. There are three centers within CMS: the Center for Beneficiary Choices, the Center for Medicare Management, and the Center for Medicaid and State Operations. Current Medicare regulations are available on the web site, as are many publications, including those about health care plans. Health care professionals who have been declared ineligible to receive Medicare and Medicaid reimbursements are listed at the web site www.defaulteddocs.dhhs.gov

ConsumerLab.com
333 Mamaroneck Avenue
White Plains, NY 10605
(914) 722-9149   e-mail: info@consumerlab.com   www.consumerlab.com

This independent laboratory tests the quality and potency of nutritional supplements and posts the results on the web site. General information is available free; complete reviews require subscription fee, $15.95. A single review is available for $5.25.

Federation of State Medical Boards (FSMB)
Federation Place
400 Fuller Wiser Road, Suite 300
Euless, TX 76039
(817) 868-4000   FAX (817) 868-4098
e-mail: alpp@fsmb.org   www.fsmb.org

A membership organization consisting of all state medical boards, this organization influences the role and policy of the boards. The web site has a consumer corner that describes the role of state boards in licensing and regulating physicians. The web site has a database of physicians who have been disciplined. A brochure "What is a State Medical Board?" is available to consumers. Free

HerbMed
www.herbmed.org

This web site provides scientific information on the medicinal use of herbs, including preparations, how they work, and warnings about their use.

National Center for Complementary and Alternative Medicine (NCCAM)
National Institutes of Health (NIH)
PO Box 8218
Silver Spring, MD 20907-8218
(888) 644-6226 (V/TT)   (301) 231-7537, extension 5
FAX (301) 495-4957   nccam.nih.gov

Conducts biomedical research in complementary and alternative medical practices. Disseminates information about complementary, alternative and unconventional medicine through toll-free telephone service, fact sheets, and information packets. Publishes quarterly newsletter, "Complementary and Alternative Medicine at the NIH," free. Also available on the web site.

National Committee for Quality Assurance (NCQA)
2000 L Street, NW, Suite 500
Washington, DC 20036
(888) 275-7585   (202) 955-3500   FAX (202) 955-3599
www.ncqa.org

An organization that evaluates and accredits health care plans so that consumers may have the information to make informed decisions about choosing a health care plan. NCQA will tell consumers whether a specific plan is accredited and provide a summary of the evaluation report. Summaries also appear on the NCQA web site.

Physicians Who Care
www.hmopage.org

This organization espouses private medical practice. The web site, written by physicians, provides information about HMOs and pending legislation that affects them. Provides a list of questions to ask your HMO.

Public Citizen Health Research Group
1600 20th Street, NW
Washington, DC 20009
(202) 588-1000   www.citizen.org

The Health Research Group promotes systemic changes in health care policy based on the research it conducts. It provides information on drugs, medical devices, doctors, and hospitals. The web site provides a list of publications and summaries of some reports.

Rosenthal Center for Complementary and Alternative Medicine
Columbia University
cpmcnet.columbia.edu/dept/rosenthal/cancer/info/choosing

This site offers fact sheets on choosing complementary and alternative medicines. May be downloaded. Free

Alternative Medicine: Expanding Medical Horizons
Superintendent of Documents
PO Box 371954
Pittsburgh, PA 15250-7954
(866) 512-1800   (202) 512-1800   FAX (202) 512-2250
e-mail: gpoaccess@gpo.gov   www.access.gpo.gov

This report by researchers and practitioners examines the status of complementary and alternative medicine in the U.S. $32.00

American Cancer Society's Guide to Complementary and Alternative Cancer Methods
American Cancer Society (ACS)
NCICFUL
PO Box 102454
Atlanta, GA 30368
(800) 227-2345   www.cancer.org

This book reviews dietary supplements such as vitamins, minerals and herbs, and therapies such as diets and alternative treatments. Provides information on insurance coverage and safety and offers ACS guidelines. Hardcover, $26.95; softcover, $19.95.

The Best Medicine: How to Choose the Top Doctors, the Top Hospitals, and the Top Treatments
by Robert Arnot
Addison-Wesley-Longman Publishing Company

This book discusses common operations, procedures, and chronic diseases. For each operation or procedure, the risks and alternatives are described and suggestions are made for choosing a physician and hospital. Out of print

Checkup on Health Insurance Choices
Agency for Healthcare Research and Quality Publications Clearinghouse
PO Box 8547
Silver Spring, MD 20907
(800) 358-9295   (888) 586-6340 (TT)   e-mail: info@ahrq.gov
www.ahrq.gov

This brochure describes health, disability, and long term care insurance; provides checklists and worksheet; and defines health insurance terms. Free

Choosing and Using a Health Plan
Agency for Healthcare Research and Quality Publications Clearinghouse
PO Box 8547
Silver Spring, MD 20907-8547
(800) 358-9295   (888) 586-6340 (TT)   e-mail: info@ahrq.gov
www.ahrq.gov

This booklet provides a basic explanation of different types of health plans and how to compare them. Available in English and Spanish. Free. Also available at the web site by clicking on "Consumer Health."

A Consumer Guide for Getting and Keeping Health Insurance
healthinsuranceinfo.net

Written by the Georgetown University Institute for Health Care Research and Policy, consumer guides are available for each state and the District of Columbia. Updated periodically as changes in federal and state policy occur.

Directory of Physicians in the United States
American Medical Association (AMA)
PO Box 930876
Atlanta, GA 31193
(800) 621-8335   (312) 464-5000   www.ama-assn.org

This directory lists all of the physicians in the U.S., both alphabetically and by geographic area. Includes information about education and training, type of medical practice, and certification. $695.00 plus $19.95 shipping and handling. It is possible to obtain the same information about physicians or to locate a certain type of physician on the AMA web site.

Doctor Shopping: How to Choose the Right Doctor for You and Your Family
by Hal Alpiar
Health Information Press
4727 Wilshire Boulevard, Suite 300
Los Angeles, CA 90010
(800) 633-7467   FAX (800) 633-6556
e-mail: info@hipbooks.com   medicalbookstore.com

This book recommends techniques for choosing a physician. Defines various medical specialties and describes how they differ. Includes checklists for evaluating physicians and health care facilities. $14.95 plus $6.95 shipping and handling

FDA Guide to Choosing Medical Treatments
www.fda.gov/oashi/aids/fdaguide.html

Reviews some of the claims and frauds associated with alternative treatments and suggests guidelines for evaluating such treatments. Available on the web site only.

Health Care Choices for Today's Consumers
by Marc S. Miller (ed.)
John Wiley and Sons
1 Wiley Drive
Somerset, NJ 08875
(800) 225-5945   (732) 469-4400   www.wiley.com

This book provides an overview of consumers' medical rights, health insurance, primary care, and hospitalization. Separate chapters describe the special needs of women, elders, and parents. $17.95

Improving Health Care Quality: A Guide for Patients and Families
Agency for Healthcare Research and Quality Publications Clearinghouse
PO Box 8547
Silver Spring, MD 20907
(800) 358-9295   (888) 586-6340 (TT)   e-mail: info@ahrq.gov
www.ahrq.gov

This booklet lists organizations, web sites, and phone numbers that can help individuals measure health care quality. Free. Also available on the web site.

The Intelligent Patient's Guide to the Doctor-Patient Relationship
by Barbara M. Korsch and Caroline Harding
Oxford University Press
2001 Evans Road
Cary, NC 27513
(800) 451-7556   FAX (919) 677-1303
e-mail: orders@oup-usa.org   www.oup-usa.org

This book suggests strategies that individuals can use to maximize their relationships with physicians. It also examines issues such as hospitalization and getting the most out of managed care. $12.95

Medicare & You
Centers for Medicare and Medicaid Services (CMS)
formerly Health Care Financing Administration (HCFA)
7500 Security Boulevard
Baltimore, MD 21244
(800) 633-4227   (410) 786-3000   www.hcfa.gov
www.medicare.gov

This booklet provides basic information about Medicare including eligibility, enrollment, coverage, and options. Free. Available in English and Spanish in print and audiocassette; in English in large print and braille. Also available on the web site.

Now You Have a Diagnosis--What's Next?
Agency for Healthcare Research and Quality Publications Clearinghouse
PO Box 8547
Silver Spring, MD 20907
(800) 358-9295   (888) 586-6340 (TT)   e-mail: info@ahrq.gov
www.ahrq.gov

This booklet discusses how to find and use reliable health care information to evaluate the risks and benefits of treatments. Available in English and Spanish. Free. Also available on the web site.

PDR for Herbal Medicines
Medical Economics Company
PO Box 10689
Des Moines, IA 50336-0689
(888) 859-8053   FAX (515) 284-6714

This reference book provides information about the most commonly used herbal medicines, including information about dosages. $59.95 plus $7.95 shipping and handling

Physicians Disciplined for Sex-Related Offenses
Public Citizen Health Research Group
1600 20th Street, NW
Washington, DC 20009
(202) 588-1000   www.citizen.org

This book reports the findings of a study which reveals that many physicians disciplined for sex-related offenses continue to practice medicine. $15.00 plus $3.00 shipping and handling

Public Citizen Health Research Group Health Letter
Public Citizen Health Research Group
1600 20th Street, NW
Washington, DC 20009
(202) 588-1000   www.citizen.org

A monthly newsletter with information about health issues such as quality of care, insurance, questionable doctors and hospitals, managed care and the recalls of drugs, devices and consumer products. $18.00. Back issues are available for $3.00 each. Membership in Public Citizen at the $35.00 level includes the "Health Letter" as well as "Public Citizen News."

Questionable Doctors
Public Citizen Health Research Group
1600 20th Street, NW
Washington, DC 20009
(202) 588-1000   www.citizen.org

This book lists the names of doctors disciplined by either state medical boards or federal agencies. National version on CD-ROM, $400.00 plus $7.50 shipping and handling; individual state information within a regional volume, $20.00 plus $3.50 shipping and handling. A summary of this report appears on the web site.

Resolution of Consumer Disputes in Managed Care: Insights from an Interdisciplinary Roundtable
American Bar Association Commission on Legal Problems of the Elderly
740 15th Street, NW
Washington, DC 20005
(202) 662-8690   FAX (202) 662-8698
e-mail: abaelderly@abanet.org   www.abanet.org/elderly

This book explores critical issues between consumers and managed care plans, such as grievances and appeals. $18.95 plus $3.95 shipping and handling

The Savvy Medical Consumer
by Charles B. Inlander and the staff of the People's Medical Society
People's Medical Society
462 Walnut Street
Allentown, PA 18102
(800) 624-8773   FAX (610) 770-0607   www.peoplesmed.org

This book provides advice on how to take control of your own medical care. It discusses how to choose a health maintenance organization, avoiding unnecessary tests, and selecting the best insurance plan. $10.95

The Scientific Review of Alternative Medicine and Aberrant Medical Practices
Prometheus Books
59 John Glenn Drive
Amherst, NY 14228
(800) 421-0351   (716) 691-0133
e-mail: marketing@prometheusbooks.com
www.prometheusbooks.com

This quarterly journal evaluates the effectiveness of various alternative medicine therapies. Individuals, $60.00; institutions, $100.00

Second Opinions: Stories of Intuition and Choice in the Changing World of Medicine
by Jerome Groopman
Viking/Penguin Putnam
375 Hudson Street
New York, NY 10014
(800) 788-6262   www.penguinputnam.com

Written by a physician, this book uses personal stories to indicate how second opinions saved the live of a variety of patients, including the author's infant son. Hardcover, $24.95; softcover, $14.00

Working with Your Doctor: Getting the Healthcare You Deserve
by Nancy Keene
O'Reilly and Associates
101 Morris Street
Sebastopol, CA 95472
(800) 998-9938   (707) 829-0515
e-mail: order@oreilly.com   www.patientcenters.com

This book provides suggestions for finding and communicating with physicians, asking about medical tests and treatments, and advocating for quality health care. $15.95 plus $4.50 shipping and handling

Wrongful Death
by Sandra M. Gilbert
W. W. Norton & Company
Keystone Industrial Park
Scranton, PA 18512
(800) 223-4830   FAX (800) 458-6515
www.wwnorton.com

Written by a woman whose husband died after routine prostate surgery, this book examines her shock and grief and the decision to sue the hospital for medical negligence. Hardcover, $22.50; softcover, $13.00; plus $4.00 shipping and handling.

Your Guide to Choosing Quality Health Care
Agency for Healthcare Research and Quality Publications Clearinghouse
PO Box 8547
Silver Spring, MD 20907-8547
(800) 358-9295   (888) 586-6340 (TT)   e-mail: info@ahrq.gov
www.ahrq.gov

This workbook offers information on choosing a health plan, physician, treatments, hospital, and long term care. Suggests questions to ask in each category. Free

ASKING THE RIGHT QUESTIONS
ABOUT MEDICAL TESTS AND PROCEDURES

Physicians often recommend medical procedures that patients are unfamiliar with. Not only should wise medical consumers ask the physician questions about the procedure and seek second opinions (and third, if necessary), but they should also search the medical literature for information about the success rate and complications that arise from the procedures. While drugs are regulated by the Food and Drug Administration, surgical procedures are not regulated by any government agency, although they may be certified by an accrediting organization.

Many individuals feel that it is better to take some type of action, even if the outcome is uncertain, rather than to let a medical condition take its natural course. This attitude undoubtedly contributes to the large number of unnecessary surgeries performed annually. The predisposition to do something rather than do nothing may incur unnecessary risks. Physicians themselves admit that there is no scientific basis for much of modern medical treatment (see, for example, Grimes: 1993). Given a lack of scientific evidence that many procedures are valuable, medical consumers should be cautious prior to agreeing to any procedure.

DIAGNOSTIC TESTS

In general, diagnostic tests are not regulated by any government agency. Most equipment is not inspected, and personnel who carry out the tests are not certified by any government agency.

You should question the purpose of any diagnostic test. If the knowledge that you have a certain condition will not result in a therapy that will cure or control the condition, is it worth it to undergo the procedure? The answer to this question is specific to the individual and the condition. In some cases, knowing that you have a disease that is genetic may help you to decide whether to have children and how to plan for your life. In other situations, the information may be more academic than practical, and you may decide the test is not valuable or worth any potential risks.

Before agreeing to any diagnostic tests, you should ask about the chances of the tests yielding false negative or false positive results. Especially with invasive tests, you should also ask about the risks of complications, such as the possibility of a colonoscopy perforating the colon or causing infections. It is possible that exposure to x-rays may result in cancer years later; therefore, you should agree to x-rays only when absolutely necessary and should learn about the amount of radiation you will be exposed to. Try to find the facility that uses the least amount of radiation to carry out the procedure.

The accuracy of diagnostic tests depends on a number of factors, including the equipment used to perform and analyze the test and the competence of the personnel performing and interpreting the test. Not only is it possible to receive another person's test results, but in many instances different laboratories report vastly different results based on an analysis of the same test. (See Chapter 10, p. 184, for an example of radiologists' interpretations of mammograms.) Therefore, if the test results do not jibe with your symptoms, you should ask to have the tests analyzed by another laboratory and have the test repeated.

It is not uncommon for unnecessary medical tests to be ordered by physicians in order to protect themselves against malpractice suits. On the other hand, physicians who work in managed care settings are financially rewarded for keeping the costs of medical care down and therefore are less likely to order tests.

In cases where tests are crucial, patients are put at greater risk if appropriate tests are not performed. Some tests are invasive and carry serious risks of complications. It is not unheard of for physicians to pressure patients into submitting to tests by scaring them or lying to them about the need for the tests. Heymann (1995), a physician herself, gives the following example:

> John, a young physician-in-training, explained that he had scared a patient into believing that she might die if a test was not performed because he was worried that she would not return for the test. He thought it was important for the patient to have the test and believed she wouldn't understand if he just explained why (p. 237).

Although John considered the patient's health as his primary concern, his approach exhibited a lack of understanding of his patient's fears, concerns, and life situation. His fear that she would not understand an explanation of the test is unjustified unless he first tried to explain it and found her unable to understand. Instead of frightening her into returning for the test, he should have questioned her about her fears, explained the importance of the test for her well-being, and described the procedure and any side effects, preparations, and precautions. He should have asked about issues in her family situation that presented a problem for returning to the hospital. Did she have children or an elderly relative that needed care? Did her religious or cultural beliefs cause her to reject certain types of medical procedures? By learning about the patient's individual situation, the physician would have engendered the sense that he cared about the patient and built a relationship based on trust, rather than fear. If, in fact, after a serious attempt to explain the situation to the patient, he or she is not capable of understanding, the patient should have a trusted relative or friend involved in discussing the situation and helping to explain it to the patient.

When a physician recommends a test to help diagnose a medical condition, you should be certain to ask questions concerning the purpose of the test and the details of how it is performed. You should also ask questions about tests that are routinely recommended when no symptoms are present (such as sigmoidoscopies and mammograms for individuals over 50). You should never assume that the test will cause no harm. The physician should have no problem providing a justification for the test if it is really necessary and safe.

Questions to ask the physician include:

• What is the purpose of the test?

- What will you learn that you do not already know? How will the results of the test affect my treatment options? Is this the least invasive test you can do to diagnose my condition?
- Is there anything controversial about this test?
- How many of these procedures have you performed? How often on someone with my symptoms? How often on someone in my age range?
- What are the mortality and morbidity rates for this procedure?
- Are the personnel who administer the tests and/or procedures, the equipment, and the facilities certified by the state or any professional organization?
- How many patients have had complications and what types of complications? What are the side effects?
- How long will the test take?
- What type of discomfort does the test cause? If it is painful, what can be done to reduce the pain? How will I feel during the test and after it? Will I be able to drive myself home after the test?
- What types of preparations are required? Do I have to discontinue any current medications? Are there any restrictions on my diet?
- How reliable is the test?
- What percentage of people in my age range have positive results?
- What are the rates of false positive or false negative results? (Many physicians will not know the answers to these statistical questions, but will come up with a round number. Ask for the source of the answer provided so that you can check it out yourself.)
- What will be the likely course of my condition if I wait to have the test?
- What are the alternatives?
- Will insurance cover the cost of the test?

If you decide to have the test, ask the physician when the results of the test will be available and to call you with the results. If you have not heard from the physician by the expected time, phone the office. Make certain that the tests are actually read and interpreted by the physician and not just filed away in your medical chart. Always obtain a written copy of the test results. Obtaining the written results will ensure that you were given the proper information verbally. The results may also play a role when consulting with other physicians or when seeking additional opinions for a difficult diagnosis.

SURGERY AND OTHER PROCEDURES

There is no federal agency that regulates the use of new surgical techniques or procedures, although the Food and Drug Administration is required to approve new medical devices, and some of these are used in surgery. New or experimental surgery may be performed without oversight by a regulatory agency. When a new type of surgery becomes popular, some surgeons may begin performing the procedure without adequate training. In addition, there are no data available on the long term effects of the surgery when it is a new procedure. For these reasons, it is important for medical consumers to research the success rate of the procedure as well as its history. Finding out whether the surgeon has a track record performing the surgery is also imperative.

The goals of surgery and other procedures vary; they are intended to save a life, to relieve pain, or to restore physical or mental functioning (Lesser: 1991). No matter what the goal, not all cases have straightforward courses to take. In many cases, there are alternatives, some carrying more risks than others. In these cases, the medical consumer must have sufficient knowledge to judge the best course for himself or herself. At the very least, medical consumers must obtain information from the physician about benefits and risks of the procedures, likelihood of success, and the likely course of the condition if it remains untreated.

Positive outcomes of medical procedures are not a sure thing. Some procedures may not only fail to improve the medical condition but may actually cause harm. An example of such a procedure described in an article in <u>JAMA</u> (Journal of the American Medical Association) is optic nerve decompression surgery. The Ischemic Optic Neuropathy Decompression Trial Research Group (1995) found that patients who received careful follow-up alone were more likely to recover spontaneously from nonarteritic anterior ischemic optic neuropathy than patients who received optic nerve decompression surgery. The surgical group was more likely to have significantly decreased visual acuity than the follow-up group. Prior to the publication of this article, the surgical procedure had been performed for patients with this condition, based on inadequate research methodologies of studies that had reported benefits of the procedure. The Ischemic Optic Neuropathy Decompression Trial Research Group, based on its controlled study, recommended that the procedure be abandoned.

Some patients may feel that physicians are pressuring them into having surgery. A noted cardiologist comments on physicians' use of scare tactics to pressure patients to have surgery:

> ...the more a doctor resorts to scare tactics, uses frightening terminology, and renders a dismal prognosis if some prescribed intervention is not pursued, the less credibility one should attach to his or her advice. A doctor who hangs out black crepe is either a salesperson or a charlatan who has never outgrown the infantile wish to play God. When obtaining a second opinion, indicate up front that whatever invasive procedures are counseled will be performed in another hospital. The physician who provides consultation must have no financial incentive whatsoever in the course of action being prescribed. (Lown: 1996, p. 68)

As Lown indicates, you should be extremely wary of physicians who use such tactics and should seek further medical consultation.

62

Surgical errors are not uncommon; however, it is difficult for medical consumers and their families to find out what really happened during surgery when a mistake was made. According to Millman (1977), who studied a number of hospitals, physicians are likely to overlook their colleagues' mistakes, because they fear reprisal. Although hospitals carry out investigations into medical cases that have become controversial, they are carried out for "educational" purposes and not for assigning blame. Families are not told of these investigations. And it is rare for a hospital to revoke admitting privileges or surgical privileges at the hospital much less take actions to revoke a medical license. One physician at a hospital Millman studied commented, "It's easier to practice medicine than to keep a driver's license" (Millman: 1977, p. 132).

Prior to consenting to surgery, you should spend time determining if the surgery is the best or only treatment for the condition, the competence of the surgeon, and the appropriateness of the hospital's facilities and equipment for performing the surgery (see Chapter 4, "Protecting Yourself in the Hospital"). You may do this in a number of ways. Doing a literature review using MEDLINE, other databases, and textbooks is the first step. Using the information obtained from this review, prepare a list of questions for the surgeon. Some general questions include the following:

- What is the purpose of the surgery? How long has this surgical procedure been in existence, and what is its success rate?
- Is this an experimental procedure?
- What are the risks? What are the benefits?
- How frequently does death occur as a result of this surgery?
- Are there alternative treatments that are equally effective? With fewer risks and side effects?
- How recently have you performed this procedure? Have you taken any courses to update your skills and learn new techniques for this surgery?
- How many times have you performed this procedure? What is your success rate?
- Do you perform all of the surgery yourself or do your associates, residents, interns, or medical students participate?
- What other professionals will be involved in the procedure - anesthesiologists, etc? What are their credentials, track records? Have they had any malpractice suits brought against them? Under what circumstances?
- Will I have the opportunity to speak with the anesthesiologist before the surgery?
- What types of complications may occur as a result of this surgery? How frequently do they occur in someone of my age, with my health status?
- Describe the techniques used for the surgery, including pre-operative preparation, post-operative care, and recuperation.

• How much blood is lost during the operation? Will I need transfusions? May I bank my own blood for transfusion?

• What drugs and anesthesia are used before, during, and after the surgery? What side effects do they cause?

• Does the hospital have up-to-date equipment for this procedure that is monitored and/or certified for proper functioning?

• What type of pain can I expect after the surgery, and what type of pain treatment do you propose?

• Do you recommend doing this surgery on an outpatient basis? If so, how long will I feel the effects of anesthesia? How long will I need someone to help me after the surgery?

• What are the qualifications of the personnel that work in the recovery room? What tests do they perform while I am a patient there?

• What effects do my other medical conditions have on my ability to withstand this surgery?

• Will I see you after the surgery? How can I get in touch with you? Will you be in town? If not, who is covering for you?

• How will I feel after the surgery, and how will my recovery proceed from day to day? How will I know if the discomfort I'm feeling is normal after this procedure or if I am experiencing a complication?

• What will my quality of life be like following the surgery? Will I have any permanent disabilities?

Additional questions will be specific to the particular medical condition involved. Similar questions should be asked for non-surgical procedures, whether performed on an outpatient or inpatient basis.

If the physician tells you that your condition is urgent and you must have surgery immediately, ask the consequences of waiting a week or a month. Is it likely that you will die as a result of waiting? Is the condition so far advanced that it is incurable? Is there any harm in waiting until you can get additional opinions and read about the condition so that you are satisfied that surgery is the right option for you? While there are conditions that must be treated immediately, most conditions, including cancer, will not be affected by delaying surgery for a short amount of time. After all, surgery is scheduled for the convenience of the medical personnel and is rarely performed on weekends, except in emergency situations.

Two consumers with the same clinical symptoms may opt for different treatments. For example, individuals with chronic, stable angina may react differently to the same severity of pain. Those affected should be aware that surgery to perform coronary artery bypass graft may not result in increased survival time, but it may result in relief of symptoms. Nease and colleagues (1995) studied 220 individuals with angina and found that individuals with the same level of pain opted for different outcomes. While some opted for symptom relief through surgery with the knowledge that their survival time would be shorter, others chose to live longer and endure their pain. Yet guidelines for treating angina put out by the American Heart

Association and the American College of Cardiology take into account only the physiological factors involved in the angina, not the desires of the individual patient.

Several precautions must be taken when entering a teaching hospital for surgery. When general anesthesia is administered prior to surgery, patients are unaware of what is happening in the operating room. This situation has resulted in what has been referred to as "ghost surgery," when a resident performs the surgery and the attending physician is not present. Another situation to be wary of is when procedures are recommended in order to educate the residents, rather than serving the health needs of the patients (Annas: 1988). Of course, the patient is never told the real reason for the surgery. In order to avoid this situation, be certain to ascertain that the surgeon you are dealing with will be performing the surgery; write it on the consent form in order to protect yourself.

CLINICAL TRIALS

Clinical trials are used to investigate the benefits and risks of new medical or surgical treatments. After a proposed new treatment has been studied in the laboratory, it must be tried in human beings to ascertain if it is safe and effective. You might agree to participate in a clinical trial in order to have access to new treatments before they are available to the public. For example, an individual who has HIV (Human Immunodeficiency Virus) might agree to participate in clinical trials hoping to delay or prevent the development of AIDS (Acquired Immune Deficiency Syndrome). Some individuals who are ineligible for conventional medical care participate in clinical trials to receive free or low cost medical services. Keep in mind that many studies include both an experimental and a control group with research subjects randomly assigned and unaware which group they are in. While the experimental group receives the treatment being tested, the control group receives a placebo. Therefore, participation in clinical trials does not guarantee that you will receive a new treatment. If you do receive the experimental treatment, it may be ineffective or cause deleterious side effects. Some treatments under investigation may have "late" effects which appear only years after the initial trial.

Clinical trials are subject to a variety of regulations. If the trial is federally funded, safeguards such as review of the protocol and the study's progress are built into the research plan. An Institutional Review Board (IRB) examines proposed clinical trials that are federally funded or federally regulated. The IRB determines whether the risks of the trial are reasonable and examines the safeguards for patients. If you are considering participating in a clinical trial, ask who is sponsoring it and who reviews and approves its methods. Ask how the study data and patient safety are monitored and where the results will be reported.

Before you enter into a clinical trial, you will be asked to sign an "informed consent" form which has been approved by the IRB. The IRB decides whether potential side effects are adequately revealed in the consent form. The IRB is meant to provide protection for individuals who enter research studies, but IRB decisions are sometimes erroneous. Occasionally, large medical research institutions have been halted in their federally funded research due to serious harm or even death of a participant, although this situation is relatively rare.

Before you give your "informed consent," you should ask the following questions:

- What is the purpose of this clinical trial?
- What kinds of tests and treatments will I undergo?
- Will I have to be hospitalized during the trial?
- What are the potential side effects?
- How will my confidentiality be protected?
- Is the treatment free? Will there be any expenses?
- What are my responsibilities during the trial? How will they affect my daily life?
- What are my treatment alternatives if I choose not to participate?

Consent forms may be difficult to understand. Ask a physician, nurse, or other health care professional to explain the terms or technical language that you don't understand. After reading the consent form, you may decide to refuse to take part in the trial. If you agree, you may choose to leave the trial at any time. If you should withdraw, your decision cannot be held against you. Make certain that the consent form clearly states your rights to refuse further participation and to withdraw from the trial at any time.

Be certain that you understand the terms that are used to describe the methods used in clinical trials. "Randomization" describes a research method in which patients with similar characteristics (symptoms, degree of disease) are randomly assigned to groups that receive different treatments. In "blind" trials, patients do not know which treatment they have received. This is supposed to remove any bias that the patients have about the value of one treatment over another. In a "double-blind" study, neither the patients nor the researchers know which patients are receiving the experimental treatment and which the placebo. Placebos are substances which have the appearance of the drug being studied but in reality have no treatment value; they are used to compare the effectiveness of the experimental treatment with the traditional treatment or no treatment. "Controls" are subjects who receive the standard treatment or no treatment for the condition under study. The results of treatment with new medications or methods may then be compared with the results of standard treatment. It is unethical for subjects to be given a placebo if there is an effective treatment for the disease.

Clinical trials are reviewed regularly. If a particular treatment is reported to be markedly better than others, the trial is halted and all the subjects are given the opportunity to receive it. For example, an international study of 1,900 patients with HIV was ended ahead of schedule when it was discovered that those patients receiving a drug called lamivudine (3TC; Epivir) along with other standard anti-AIDS drugs, such as AZT, ddI, or ddC, fared much better than those in a control group who received only the standard anti-AIDS drugs (Knox: 1996). If a treatment is found to be harmful, ineffective, or causes dangerous side effects, the trial is stopped.

To find out about clinical trials, contact the National Institutes of Health or specific programs such as the National Cancer Institute (NCI) or the American Foundation for AIDS Research (AmFAR). PDQ, the National Cancer Institute's computerized database, provides information about clinical trials on the Internet, through e-mail, and by telephone request to the Cancer Information Center (see "ORGANIZATIONS" section below). AmFAR publishes a directory of clinical trials, updated twice a year (see "PUBLICATIONS" section below).

The online resource, Center Watch Clinical Trials Listing Service (www.centerwatch.com) lists clinical trials by general field, such as endocrinology, ophthalmology, cardiology, etc.

References

Annas, George J.
1988 Judging Medicine Clifton, NJ: Humana Press
Grimes, David A.
1993 "Technology Follies" JAMA 269:23(June 16):3030-3033
Heymann, Jody
1995 Equal Partners: A Physician's Call for a New Spirit of Medicine Boston, MA: Little, Brown and Company
The Ischemic Optic Neuropathy Decompression Trial Research Group
1995 "Optic Nerve Decompression Surgery for Nonarteritic Anterior Ischemic Optic Neuropathy (NAION) Is Not Effective and May Be Harmful" JAMA 273:8(February 22):625-632
Knox, Richard A.
1996 "Success of a New AIDS Treatment Brings Study to Early End" Boston Globe July 24
Lesser, Harry
1991 "The Patient's Right to Information" pp. 150-160 in Margaret Brazier and Mary Lobjoit (eds.) Protecting the Vulnerable: Autonomy and Consent in Health Care London and New York: Routledge
Lown, Bernard
1996 The Lost Art of Healing Boston, MA: Houghton Mifflin Company
Millman, Marcia
1977 The Unkindest Cut New York, NY: William Morrow and Company
Nease, Robert F., Jr. et al.
1995 "Variation in Patient Utilities for Outcome of the Management of Chronic Stable Angina: Implications for Clinical Practice Guidelines" JAMA 273:15(April 19):1185-1190

ORGANIZATIONS

Agency for Healthcare Research and Quality (AHRQ)
2101 East Jefferson Street, Suite 501
Rockville, MD 20852
(301) 594-1364   e-mail: info@ahrq.gov   www.ahrq.gov

A federal agency that funds research studies on effectiveness of medical treatments, economic aspects of health care policy, and quality of care. Publishes monthly newsletter, "Research Activities." Free. Newsletter and reports also available on the web site.

American College of Surgeons
633 North Saint Clair Street
Chicago, IL 60611
(312) 202-5000   FAX (312) 202-5001
e-mail: postmaster@facs.org   www.facs.org

A professional organization for surgeons, this group publishes a series of pamphlets for medical consumers, including "It's Your Choice," "Should You Seek Consultation? (Second Opinion)," "Giving Your Informed Consent," "What Will Your Operation Cost?" and "Who Should Do Your Operation?" Single copy, free. Also available on the web site.

American Foundation for AIDS Research (AmFAR)
120 Wall Street, 13th floor
New York, NY 10005
(800) 392-6327   (212) 806-1600
FAX (212) 806-1601   e-mail: amfar@amfar.org   www.amfar.org

Funds basic biomedical research; operates the Community-Based Clinical Trials Network which enables physicians across the country to enroll patients in trials of new drugs and new therapies; and funds education for AIDS prevention. Publishes "The AMFAR Report" and "The AmFAR Newsletter."

Association for Patient-Oriented Research (APOR)
c/o Jules Hirsch
Rockefeller University
New York, NY 10021-6399
e-mail: apor@amcmail.vanderbilt.edu   www.apor.org

An organization founded by physicians to encourage more clinical research.

Cancer Liaison Program
Office of Special Health Issues
Food and Drug Administration (FDA)
5600 Fishers Lane, HF-12, Room 9-49
Rockville, MD 20857
(888) 463-6332   (301) 827-4460   FAX (301) 443-4555
e-mail: OSHI@oc.fda.gov   www.fda.gov/oashi/cancer/cancer.html

Informs cancer patients and their families about the FDA drug approval process, cancer clinical trials, and access to investigational therapies.

Centers for Medicare and Medicaid Services (CMS)
formerly Health Care Financing Administration (HCFA)
7500 Security Boulevard
Baltimore, MD 21244
(800) 633-4227   (410) 786-3000   www.hcfa.gov
www.medicare.gov

In addition to administering Medicare and Medicaid, CMS regulates all laboratory tests (except research).

Center Watch Clinical Trials Listing Service
www.centerwatch.com

Lists clinical trials by general field, such as endocrinology, ophthalmology, etc. Lists new FDA approvals. Links to other health sites on the Internet.

National Cancer Institute (NCI)
Physician Data Query (PDQ)
CancerNet
CANCERLIT
LiveHelp
31 Center Drive MSC 2580
Building 31, Room 10A03
Bethesda, MD 20892
(800) 422-6237   (800) 332-8615 (TT)   FAX (301) 402-5874
CancerFax (800) 624-2511   e-mail: cancermail@cips.nci.nih.gov
cancer.gov

The National Cancer Institute supports basic and clinical research investigations into the causes, prevention, and cure for cancer. The PDQ database provides up-to-date information on cancer prevention, screening, clinical trials, treatments, and care. PDQ is available on the Internet through CancerNet, which also contains fact sheets and publications, CancerNet news, and CANCERLIT abstracts and citations. CancerFax provides access by fax machine to information statements from the PDQ Database, CANCERLIT citations and abstracts, and fact sheets on cancer topics. LiveHelp is a pilot program that provides live, online assistance from an NCI Information Specialist; available Monday-Friday, 12:00 to 4:00 p.m., Eastern Time. Most information is also available in Spanish. Calling the "800" phone number listed above connects with the regional center closest to you, which can provide information about the resources described above as well as local resources.

National Institutes of Health Consensus Program
PO Box 2577
Kensington, MD 20891
(888) 644-2667   FAX (301) 816-2494
e-mail: consensus_statements@nih.gov
consensus.nih.gov

Sponsors conferences that produce consensus statements on the effectiveness, risks, and clinical applications of biomedical technology. Consensus statements on subjects such as breast cancer screening, kidney dialysis, impotence, epilepsy, pain management, and osteoporosis are available on the web site.

National Organization for Rare Disorders (NORD)
100 Rt. 37, PO Box 8923
New Fairfield, CT 06812-8923
(800) 999-6673   (203) 746-6518   (203) 746-6927 (TT)
FAX (203) 746-6481   e-mail: orphan@rarediseases.org
www.rarediseases.org

Federation of voluntary health organizations that serves individuals with rare or "orphan" diseases. Maintains a confidential patient networking program for individuals and family members who have been diagnosed with a rare disorder. Membership, $30.00. Reprints of articles on rare diseases available from the NORD Rare Disease Database for $7.50 per copy; abstracts available free on web site. Publishes newsletter, "Orphan Disease Update," three times a year; free.

People's Medical Society
462 Walnut Street
Allentown, PA 18102
(800) 624-8773   FAX (610) 770-0607   www.peoplesmed.org

This consumer health advocacy organization publishes books, health bulletins, and fact sheets on many aspects of medical care. Membership, $20.00, includes bimonthly "People's Medical Society Newsletter." The list of publications, "Health Library Catalog," is free.

YourSurgery.com
yoursurgery.com

This multimedia site uses simple diagrams and animation to show common surgical procedures.

PUBLICATIONS

AIDS/HIV Clinical Trial Handbook
American Foundation for AIDS Research (AmFAR)
120 Wall Street, 13th floor
New York, NY 10005
(800) 392-6327   (212) 806-1600
FAX (212) 806-1601   e-mail: amfar@amfar.org   www.amfar.org

This booklet discusses the benefits and risks of participation in clinical trials. Free

Be Informed: Questions to Ask Your Doctor Before You Have Surgery
Agency for Healthcare Research and Quality Publications Clearinghouse
PO Box 8547
Silver Spring, MD 20907-8547
(800) 358-9295   (888) 586-6340 (TT)   e-mail: info@ahrq.org
www.ahrq.gov

This brochure poses 12 questions to ask physicians before choosing to have elective surgery. Covers issues such as benefits and risks, recovery time, and possible alternatives to surgery. Available in English and Spanish. Free. Also available on the web site by clicking on "Consumer Health."

Cancer Clinical Trials: Experimental Treatments and How They Can Help You
by Robert Finn
O'Reilly and Associates
101 Morris Street
Sebastopol, CA 95472
(800) 998-9938   (707) 829-0515
e-mail: order@oreilly.com   www.patientcenters.com

This book compares information on experimental treatment options to standard treatment protocols. $14.95 plus $4.50 shipping and handling

The Consumer's Legal Guide to Today's Health Care
by Stephen L. Isaacs and Ava C. Schwartz
Houghton Mifflin Company, Boston, MA

This book describes patients' legal rights regarding treatment options, insurance (including Medicare and medical supplemental insurance), long term care, the right to die, as well as the need for a lawyer. Out of print.

Equal Partners: A Physician's Call for a New Spirit of Medicine
by Jody Heymann
Little, Brown and Company, Boston, MA

In this book, a physician whose experiences with severe brain seizures changed her perception of medical care discusses her personal encounters as well as her suggestions for a better form of medicine. Out of print.

Good Operations, Bad Operations
by Charles B. Inlander
Viking/Penguin, New York, NY

This book provides guidelines for choosing surgeons and specialists, including a surgical checklist. Descriptions of 100 of the most commonly performed diagnostic and surgical procedures include mortality and morbidity rates, complications and possible side effects, alternatives, and whether there is anything controversial about the procedure. Includes glossary and resource list. Out of print

HIV/AIDS Treatment Directory
American Foundation for AIDS Research (AmFAR)
120 Wall Street, 13th floor
New York, NY 10005
(800) 392-6327   (212) 806-1600
FAX (212) 806-1601   e-mail: amfar@amfar.org   www.amfar.org

This semi-annual publication includes information about the latest prevention strategies and treatments, drug assistance programs, drug trials that are actively seeking participants, and other resources such as hotlines and community based treatment programs. Individuals, $55.00; physicians/institutions, $125.00. Individuals with HIV/AIDS who cannot afford a subscription may obtain a free copy by calling the CDC National Prevention Information Network at (800) 458-5231.

Informed Consent: Participation in Genetic Research Studies
Genetic Alliance
4301 Connecticut Avenue, NW, Suite 404
Washington, DC 20008
(800) 336-4363   (202) 966-5557   FAX (202) 966-8553
e-mail: info@geneticalliance.org   www.geneticalliance.org

This booklet is designed to help individuals decide whether or not to participate in a genetic research clinical trial. $1.00

Johns Hopkins Medical Handbook and Directory
Random House
400 Hahn Road
Westminster, MD 21157
(800) 733-3000   (410) 848-1900   FAX (410) 386-7013
www.randomhouse.com

This book describes 100 major medical conditions seen in people over age 50. Discusses symptoms, diagnosis, and treatment. Includes listings of teaching hospitals, treatment centers, and support organizations. $39.95 plus $5.50 shipping and handling

Lab Tests and Diagnostic Procedures
by Cynthia C. Chernecky and Barbara J. Berger (eds.)
Reed Elsevier Health Sciences
11830 Westline Industrial Park
St. Louis, MO 63146
(800) 545-2522   FAX (800) 568-5136
www.harcourthealth.com

This clinical laboratory/diagnostic reference book provides information for all age groups, describes symptoms and signs of overdose, and includes suggestions for patient and family teaching. $34.95

NORD Resource Guide
National Organization for Rare Disorders (NORD)
100 Rt. 37, PO Box 8923
New Fairfield, CT 06812-8923
(800) 999-6673   (203) 746-6518   (203) 746-6927 (TT)
FAX (203) 746-6481   e-mail: orphan@rarediseases.org
www.rarediseases.org

This directory lists organizations that support individuals with rare diseases and disabilities. $45.00 plus $5.00 shipping and handling

The Patient's Guide to Medical Tests
by Faculty Members of the Yale University School of Medicine
Barry L. Zaret et al. (eds.)
Houghton Mifflin
181 Ballardvale Street, PO Box 7050
Wilmington, MA 01887
(800) 225-3362   FAX (800) 634-7568   www.hmco.com

After describing screening, diagnostic imaging and laboratory testing in general, this book discusses specific tests conducted on the organs and systems of the body and for conditions such as diabetes, hypertension, HIV/AIDS, infectious and genetic diseases. Information is provided on preparation, procedure, interpretation, advantages, and disadvantages of each test and what the next step might be. Includes discussion of patients' rights and informed consent. $40.00 plus 18% shipping and handling

The Patient's Guide to Medical Tests: Everything You Need to Know About the Tests Your Doctor Prescribes
by Joseph C. Segen and Joseph Stauffer
Facts on File, Inc.
132 West 31st Street, 17th Floor
New York, NY 10001
(800) 322-8755, extension 4228   FAX (800) 678-3633
www.factsonfile.com

This book lists common medical tests, including their purpose; patient preparation; what procedures will be carried out; a reference range of values for persons free of the condition and an explanation of any abnormal values observed; the cost of the test; and comments about risks or precautions associated with the test. Includes a glossary and a list of medical abbreviations and symbols. $40.00 plus $4.00 shipping and handling

Patient's Guide to Surgery
by Edward L. Bradley
University of Pennsylvania Press
PO Box 4836, Hampden Station
Baltimore, MD 21211-0836
(800) 445-9880   (215) 898-6261

This book offers suggestions on choosing a surgeon, including questions to ask prospective candidates. It describes anesthesia choices and post-surgical pain control techniques. Includes information on 34 common operations, such as the purpose of the surgery, non-surgical alternatives, surgical techniques, risks, and what to expect after surgery. $27.50 plus $4.75 shipping and handling

The Surgery Book: An Illustrated Guide to 73 of the Most Common Operations
by Robert M. Youngson
St. Martin's Press
c/o VHPS
16365 James Madison Highway
Gordonville, VA 22942
(800) 321-9299   www.stmartins.com

Written by a physician, this book describes conditions that require surgery, pre-surgical diagnostic tests, the operating room and staff, surgical techniques, post-surgical effects, and long term effects. $17.95

Taking Part in Clinical Trials: What Cancer Patients Need to Know
Cancer Information Center, National Cancer Institute (NCI)
31 Center Drive MSC 2580
Building 31, Room 10A03
Bethesda, MD 20892
(800) 422-6237   (800) 332-8615 (TT)   FAX (301) 402-5874
CancerFax (800) 624-2511   e-mail: cancermail@cips.nci.nih.gov
cancer.gov

This booklet provides the pros and cons of taking part in clinical trials. Free. Also available on the web site.

When You Need An Operation
American College of Surgeons
633 North Saint Clare Street
Chicago, IL 60611
(312) 202-5000   FAX (312) 202-5001
e-mail: postmaster@facs.org   www.facs.org

This brochure answers questions about elective surgery, including topics such as second opinions, evaluating physicians' credentials, and informed consent. Free. Also available on the web site.

Who Cares: Sources of Information About Health Care Products and Services
Federal Trade Commission
600 Pennsylvania Avenue, NW, Room H-130
Washington, DC 20580
(877) 382-4357   FAX (202) 326-2572
e-mail: publications@ftc.gov   www.ftc.gov

This booklet lists federal, state, and private resources for information on subjects such as medical treatments, hearing aids, prescription drugs, and nursing facilities. Free. Also available on the web site.

Chapter 4

PROTECTING YOURSELF IN THE HOSPITAL

Many patients have described their experiences in hospitals as extremely regimented and repressive, akin to being a prisoner. Upon entering a hospital, patients are stripped of their own clothing and given a hospital johnny, issued an identification bracelet, required to eat at predetermined times, and to submit to tests that are scheduled for the convenience of the hospital staff. This type of situation would fit Goffman's (1961) description of a "total institution," where all vestiges of individuality are taken away, and the institution attempts to control all aspects of daily life.

A study of the factors that contributed to surgical patients' conformity or deviance regarding hospital rules and regulations found that elderly and less educated patients were the most likely to conform (Lorber: 1975). Patients who were labeled "problem patients" by doctors and nurses because they failed to conform received more time and attention from the staff.

The hospital's attempt to gain complete control over the patient begins when the patient first enters. Before being "admitted," patients are required to sign general consent forms indicating that they are entering the hospital voluntarily and that they give consent for a broad array of procedures related to diagnosis, treatment, biopsy, and surgery (Heymann: 1995). The broad scope of the consent form gives the hospital and its staff virtual free rein over the patient's body.

By asking for a copy of the form prior to entering the hospital, you will be able to read it thoroughly without an admitting clerk pressuring you to sign it. Make the changes you feel are necessary, deleting and adding conditions. When you arrive at the hospital, point out the changes you have made. You may need to negotiate on some of these points for the hospital to agree to your conditions. Remember that consent forms are designed to protect the hospital and medical staff, not the patient. Understand what you are signing and refuse to consent to blanket statements in order to protect yourself during your hospital stay.

Consent forms for specific procedures indicate possible risks incurred when undergoing a medical procedure. They also have clauses that permit hospital staff such as interns to observe and participate in the procedure. Prior to surgery or any other invasive procedure, specify on the consent form that only the expected physician may perform the procedure. Should you decide that some of the hospital's stipulations are not to your advantage, cross them out and initial them, making certain that the person who has administered the form is aware that you have made changes. You may also write in your own stipulations.

The Patient's Self-Determination Act of 1990 requires that patients be informed of their right to accept or refuse medical treatment and to have advance directives (see Chapter 5, p. 93). Most hospitals now provide patients with a copy of a "Patient's Bill of Rights," which has been developed by the American Hospital Association. This document has been criticized for addressing issues of courtesy but failing to address patients' rights (Annas: 1989).

Nash (1985), a physician, recommends that individuals who are entering a hospital keep a diary of all the tests that are performed. In addition, he suggests that hospital patients only permit their blood to be drawn once a day, even if multiple tests are to be performed.

CHOOSING A HOSPITAL

Not all hospitals are alike. Teaching hospitals are facilities where interns and residents comprise a large fraction of the house staff, while community hospitals are smaller facilities with no affiliations with medical schools. Some medical consumers may feel uncomfortable in teaching hospitals, because groups of residents and interns along with an attending physician make rounds discussing each case, often in front of the patient.

Teaching hospitals have two goals: to treat patients and to teach interns and residents. In some instances, these two goals may come into conflict. It is not uncommon for residents to carry out surgeries (presumably under the supervision of an attending physician). Medical specialty boards require that residents perform a certain number of surgeries or procedures within the given specialty. In order to meet these requirements, sometimes patients undergo surgery, unaware that the surgery has been recommended so that a resident may complete the requisite number of surgeries and that no treatment or treatment with drugs would have been effective. Some surgeries performed in teaching hospitals may be considered experimental; be certain to inquire if this is the case for surgery proposed for your condition. If the surgery is experimental, consider it very carefully before agreeing to the operation. In cases where no other treatment is available and the condition may cause serious effects if left untreated, many people will opt for the treatment. Be certain you know the possible risks of the surgery and have read all possible descriptions and evaluations of the procedure.

It is often assumed that teaching hospitals have all of the necessary equipment to perform the most sophisticated procedures. In choosing a hospital, however, you must consider the condition to be treated and base your decision upon the quality of the department that deals with that condition. The qualifications of the staff and the equipment available are two criteria you should use to make your decision. The best way to do this is to review the literature on the treatment protocols, develop a set of questions for the physician and staff, and then make up your mind about which is the best hospital for you. Many teaching hospitals put residents in charge of patient cases, presumably under the supervision of an attending (senior) physician. If you or someone you are advocating for are being treated by residents and you are concerned that the care is inadequate or ineffective, insist upon speaking with the attending physician. If this yields no satisfaction, phone your private physician for assistance. This tactic and/or transferring to another hospital has saved many a life (for example, Groopman: 2000).

It is very common to acquire an infectious disease by virtue of staying in the hospital. The incidence of these infections has increased by more than a third (36%) over the two decades between 1975 and 1995 (Reuters: 1998), probably because these infections, called nosocomial infections, are increasingly resistant to antibiotics. Often transmitted in the urinary or respiratory tract as a result of intubation in these areas, these infections may cause complications related to surgery and delay recovery; in some instances, they are fatal (Boston Women's Health Book Collective: 1992). If hospital personnel washed their hands before making physical contacts with patients, the rate of nosocomial infections would decline (Reuters: 1998). Make sure to insist that hospital staff wash their hands before touching you. Regulations require that hospital staff wear gloves when performing many procedures; insist that they do so.

A study of 31,000 records from New York hospitals revealed that, while they were hospitalized, almost one out of 25 patients suffered an adverse event (an injury from medical intervention or care rather than from disease); a third of these were due to negligence (Brennan et al.: 1991). Examples of negligence included failure or delay in diagnosis or treatment. About 50% of the adverse events were related to surgery, while drugs were also frequently involved. Elders were more likely to experience injuries due to negligence.

In many instances, choosing a hospital is connected to choosing a physician. However, it is still wise to check out the hospital before committing yourself to stay with a given physician. Phone the hospital to learn the success rate it has in treating your specific condition. Ask about the ratio of nurses to patients and the percentage of physicians who are board certified. Ask about any affiliations with medical schools.

RECEIVING TREATMENT IN THE EMERGENCY ROOM

Many Americans find themselves in the hospital emergency room when they need treatment on an urgent basis and their physician is not available. In 1999, nearly 103 million visits were made to emergency rooms. About 20 percent of noninstitutionalized individuals made at least one visit to the emergency room and seven percent made two or more visits (McCaig and Burt: 2001). Patients who are conscious and alert have the right to tell the ambulance driver the hospital they prefer, and the person who accompanies the patient may also do so. Unfortunately, recent closures and mergers of hospitals have resulted in a shortage of emergency room facilities. Emergency rooms have been forced to shut down for hours at a time because they lack the staff to treat the growing number of patients that arrive.

It is apparent that there is no time for research when an emergency is at hand. Going to a hospital where an individual has had previous positive experiences, where the patient's primary care physician practices, or where there is a reputable department that works in the required specialty area is a good way of choosing a destination.

Receiving care in the emergency room of a hospital can be very frustrating for both patients and those accompanying them. Privacy is at a minimum, and personnel often try to keep accompanying persons in the waiting room. Patients who are alert should assert their preference for having an advocate with them at all times.

Often a patient who receives treatment in the emergency room is admitted as an inpatient to the hospital. At that point, the suggestions below apply to the hospital stay.

CHOOSING AN ADVOCATE FOR YOUR HOSPITAL STAY

If possible, you should select someone that you trust to act as your advocate when you are unable to advocate for yourself. Be certain to discuss with your advocate the alternatives available and your preferences. This will ensure that your wishes are followed in the event that you are unable to communicate at a time when a crucial decision must be made. You may need to complete a health care proxy form, legally appointing your advocate. This may be especially important if the person you wish to be your advocate is not your next of kin or not related to you at all. Check with the state department of health to learn the legal requirements in your state. Many hospitals now employ patient representatives, who, despite their titles, actually represent the hospital's interests, since they are on the hospital's payroll. Do not rely on the hospital's employees instead of your own personal advocate.

AVOIDING MEDICAL ERRORS

Everyone has heard horror stories about patients who have had the wrong limb amputated or patients who died from overdosages of medication or the wrong medication. The actual number of medical errors that cause death among hospitalized patients in this country is a subject of current controversy. The Institute of Medicine (IOM) reported that as many as 98,000 deaths occur each year that are caused by medical errors that could have been prevented (Corrigan et al.: 1999). Other investigators have disputed this estimate, claiming that the number is far less. Hayward and Hofer (2001) used similar methods as the IOM study and had similar findings, even though they had originally eliminated terminally ill patients from their study. Both studies found that approximately a quarter of patient deaths had possibly been caused by medical error. Hayward and Hofer found that six percent of deaths were probably or definitely preventable. After adjusting for reviewer variability, they estimated that .5 percent of the patients would have lived three months or more cognitively intact. Thus, they concluded that roughly one patient in every 10,000 hospital admissions dies as a result of medical error.

Errors may occur due to misdiagnosis, misinterpretation of diagnostic tests, or medication errors (the wrong medicine is prescribed, two or more medications produce a harmful interaction, or the dosage is wrong). Surgical errors may be due to surgical techniques, wound infection, or post-operative bleeding. And while not all errors result in death, some may result in extended hospital stays or the need for a long recuperation period.

All patients and advocates should take precautions to prevent such adverse events. Ask as many questions as needed to be satisfied that you have received the correct diagnosis (See Chapter 3). Ask to have test results explained in detail and to see them in writing. Read the literature on treatment for the condition in order to understand possible benefits and side effects.

In an attempt to avoid medication errors, some hospitals have provided their staff with hand-held computers to enter orders for a patient's care. This method prevents misinterpretation of handwriting and helps to ensure that the orders are entered for the correct patient. Even when these precautions have been taken by the staff, it is wise to check the medications that the hospital staff brings to you, to be able to identify the medications as ones that you know have been prescribed and are safe for you. When you find an unfamiliar medication, ask what it is and who prescribed it; then contact the prescribing physician and question him or her about this medication. When you are having surgery, make certain that the surgeon operates on the proper organ, especially if it is a limb. Have the hospital staff mark which limb is to be operated on with an indelible pen.

Take a notebook to the hospital with you to record procedures, medications, and interviews. Be certain that you understand why blood samples are taken, to ensure that unnecessary duplication is not taking place. Know the medications that you should take and what they look like, so that you can check to be sure you are getting the correct drugs and dosages. Teach your advocate to fill in for you when you are not alert enough to monitor for yourself.

Some hospitals now employ a new type of physician, a hospitalist. Hospitalists are often called upon to treat patients when the primary care physician is not available or when there is a question about the diagnosis or treatment. When someone you do not know comes to examine you or ask you questions, ask the person who he or she is, their medical position, and why they have come. Be certain that this person is thoroughly familiar with your medical history in order to avoid unnecessary and duplicative tests and procedures or those that may prove harmful.

The hospital staff may feel uncomfortable with constant oversight and try to intimidate you from taking these measures, but your health and your life are at stake. Hospitals are not the only settings where medical errors may occur. Treatments provided in nursing homes, outpatient clinics, doctors' offices, and at home are also subject to errors.

ANESTHESIA AND POST-SURGICAL PAIN CONTROL

Anesthesia is used in surgery to block nerve transmissions, resulting in loss of feeling or sensation and relieving pain. The three major types of anesthesia are general, regional, and local.

General anesthesia is administered through inhaled anesthetics and intravenous injections. With general anesthesia, you are unconscious with no sensation throughout your body. Combinations of anesthetic agents are used: barbiturates, such as sodium thiopental (Pentothal) are used to slow nerve transmission; benzodiazepine, a tranquilizer that creates amnesia of surgical events; neuromuscular relaxants; and opiates, to dilute the anesthetic (Bradley: 1994). Since general anesthesia affects blood pressure, respiration, and heart rate, these functions are monitored during surgery. After surgery is completed, anesthetics are discontinued, and medications are used to reverse their effects and to diminish discomfort in the post-operative period.

Regional anesthesia, such as a spinal or an epidural block, is injected directly into the specific region where surgery will be performed, allowing you to remain conscious during the surgery. In addition, sedation is often given to reduce anxiety and induce relaxation. Pain relief may take 10 to 20 minutes after injection. The spinal block is injected into the spinal cord fluid, quickly blocking sensation below the injection site. An epidural block is injected between the vertebrae into the outer lining of the spinal cord through a catheter which is left in place to permit administration of additional anesthesia as needed. Epidural blocks are often used to provide pain relief to women during labor and delivery, because they permit the mother to feel contractions and push when needed.

Local anesthesia is injected directly into a specific area of nerves, such as those behind the eye for cataract surgery. Surface anesthesia is a type of local anesthesia that is sprayed or rubbed into the skin in the form of gel or cream.

Post-surgical pain relief may be provided in a variety of ways. Painkillers, such as morphine, are routinely given to ease pain so that patients can resume near normal mobility as soon as possible. Although some individuals fear narcotic addiction, the pain relief afforded by these drugs may enable them to recuperate more rapidly. Intravenous patient-controlled analgesia (PCA) permits the individual to control the amount of medication provided. Clinicians pre-set the dosages and frequencies in order to prevent overdosing (Walker: 1995). PCA allows patients to self-administer pain relief without calling -- and waiting -- for a nurse.

An interview with an anesthesiologist or nurse anesthetist should take place prior to surgery. It may take place by telephone, but is preferably done in person at the surgical facility. Although it is possible to request a specific anesthesiologist (if time allows), in most cases, the anesthesiologist is assigned on a rotating basis or chosen by the surgeon. You should ask who will actually administer the anesthetic and inquire about that individual's credentials.

The anesthesiologist should discuss the upcoming surgery and describe anesthesia choices, as well as their risks and benefits. Depending on the surgery, you may be able to choose one type of anesthesia over another; i.e., if you fear losing consciousness, you may request a regional anesthetic, while someone else may prefer to be completely unconscious. The anesthesiologist should obtain information about medical conditions such as diabetes, kidney or stomach disorders, sickle cell anemia, breathing problems, hypertension, or heart problems; use of medications, steroids, cigarettes, alcohol, or recreational drugs; contact lenses or false teeth; allergies to latex; and recent history of colds or flu.

If you take medications on a regular basis, you should discuss whether or not they should be taken on the day of surgery or discontinued for a specific period of time prior to surgery. Individuals are often instructed to discontinue aspirin or other anti-inflammatory drugs ten days to two weeks before surgery; if this will dramatically affect inflammation due to arthritis, a bleeding time test may be performed. This test measures the time required for a small puncture wound to stop bleeding. If it stops bleeding within a normal range (3 to 6 minutes), the daily medication regimen may be continued.

Discuss any medications you take regularly with the physician to determine when it is safe to resume taking them. Ten to twenty percent of individuals who undergo general anesthesia experience side effects such as nausea and vomiting (Bradley: 1994). Ask if there is an antinausea medication that you can take prior to surgery.

DISCHARGE FROM THE HOSPITAL

Premature discharges from the hospital may be hazardous to patients. Medicare patients who believe that they are being discharged prematurely may appeal the discharge to their state's Peer Review Organization (PRO), which monitors the quality of service provided to recipients by physicians, hospitals, nursing facilities, HMOs, and home health agencies. PROs oversee the quality of care, investigate all written complaints from patients, impose penalties for inappropriate or poor quality care, and rule on appeals.

Utilization review is used by managed care plans to reduce hospital admissions and control the length of inpatient stays through preadmission certification, second opinions for surgical procedures, and discharge planning. An appeals process is available to medical consumers and their physicians if they disagree with the review. However, in many cases, the appeals process takes too long to be helpful. It is wise to determine your health care plan's discharge policies and its appeals process before you need hospital care.

References

Annas, George J.
1989   The Rights of Patients Totowa, NJ: Humana Press

Boston Women's Health Book Collective
1992   The New Our Bodies, Our Selves New York, NY: Simon and Schuster

Bradley, Edward L.
1994   Patient's Guide to Surgery Philadelphia, PA: University of Pennsylvania Press

Brennan, Troyen et al.
1991   "Incidence of Adverse Events and Negligence in Hospitalized Patients: Results of the Harvard Medical Practice Study I" New England Journal of Medicine 324:6(February):370-77

Corrigan, Janet, Linda Kohn, and Molla Donaldson
1999   To Err is Human: Building a Safer Health System Washington, DC: National Academy Press

Goffman, Erving
1961   Asylums Garden City, NY: Anchor Books

Groopman, Jerome
2000   Second Opinions: Stories of Intuition and Choice in the Changing World of Medicine New York, NY: Viking/Penguin Putnam

Hayward, Rodney A. and Timothy P. Hofer
2001   "Estimating Hospital Deaths Due to Medical Errors" JAMA 286:4(July 25):415-420

Heymann, Jody
1995   Equal Partners: A Physician's Call for a New Spirit of Medicine Boston, MA: Little, Brown and Company

Lorber, Judith
1975   "Good Patients and Problem Patients: Conformity and Deviance in a General Hospital" Journal of Health and Social Behavior 16:2(June):213-225

McCaig, Linda F. and Catharine W. Burt
2001   "National Hospital Ambulatory Medical Care Survey: 1999 Emergency Department Summary" Advance Data from Vital and Health Statistics No. 320, June 25 Hyattsville, MD: National Center for Health Statistics

Nash, David
1985   Medical Mayhem New York, NY: Walker and Co.

Reuters
1998   "Infection Rates Rise at US Hospitals" Boston Globe March 12

Walker, Janice D.
1995   "Enhancing Physical Comfort in the Hospital" The Picker Report 3:1:(Winter):1-2, 5

ORGANIZATIONS

American Association of Nurse Anesthetists (AANA)
222 South Prospect Avenue
Park Ridge, IL 60068
(847) 692-7050   FAX (847) 692-6968
e-mail: chodson@aana.com   www.aana.com

A professional membership organization for nurse anesthetists. Accredits nurse anesthesia education programs, certifies graduates through a national examination (CRNA, Certified Registered Nurse Anesthetists), and recertifies CRNAs biennially. Publishes patient education brochures, such as "Before Anesthesia: Your Active Role Makes a Difference;" "After Anesthesia: Your Active Role Assists Your Recovery;"and "Anesthesia Options for Labor and Delivery." Available in English and Spanish. Free

American Society of Anesthesiologists (ASA)
520 North Northwest Highway
Park Ridge, IL 60068
(847) 825-5586   FAX (847) 825-1692   e-mail: mail@asahq.org
www.asahq.org

A professional membership organization for anesthesiologists. Publishes patient education brochures, such as "Know Your Anesthesiologist," "Anesthesia for Ambulatory Surgery," "When Your Child Needs Anesthesia," and "The Senior Citizen as a Patient." Single copy, free. Also available on the web site.

Health Care Choices
PO Box 21039
Columbia Circle Station, NY 10023
www.healthcarechoices.org

The web site provides physician profiles and information about hospitals, insurance plans, and specific health conditions. It includes a number of issues to address when selecting a hospital.

HealthScope
www.healthscope.org

Although the searches on this web site are limited to California facilities, there are helpful links on topics such as choosing a hospital, choosing a hospital for surgery, hospital quality checklist, and how to file a complaint on hospital care.

Hospital Select
www.hospitalselect.com

This web site provides basic information on U.S. hospitals, including size, accreditation, and frequencies of surgical procedures. Links to web sites for choosing physicians and other specialists.

Hospital Web
neuro-www2.mgh.harvard.edu/hospitalwebusa.html

Index of hospitals that have Internet home pages.

Institute for Safe Medication Practices (ISMP)
1800 Byberry Road, Suite 819
Huntington Valley, PA 19006
(215) 947-7797   FAX (215) 914-1492
e-mail: ismpinfo@ismp.org   www.ismp.org

Provides assistance to callers regarding medication errors and medication error prevention methods. Maintain reference articles covering this subject. Administers the Medication Errors Reporting Program, which enables health care professionals to report medication errors or potential errors. Web site includes information about medical alerts and links to other sites.

Joint Commission on Accreditation of Healthcare Organizations (JCAHO)
1 Renaissance Boulevard
Oakbrook Terrace, IL 60181
(630) 792-5000   FAX (630) 792-5005   www.jcaho.org

This organization provides accreditation to health care organizations including hospitals, home care, long term care, and ambulatory care facilities. The health care facilities must pay for the accreditation survey. Criteria used for accreditation evaluations are described on the web site and in JCAHO publications. JCAHO has a consumer information section on its web site, where it is possible to find the accreditation status of specific facilities. Consumers may file complaints about facilities by phoning (800) 994-6610 or e-mailing to complaint@jcaho.org. Consumer publications such as "Helping You Choose the Hospital for You" and "Helping You Choose a Quality Health Plan" are available. Single copy, free. Also available on the web site.

National Association of Hospital Hospitality Houses (NAHHH)
PO Box 18087
Asheville, NC 28814-0087
(800) 542-9730   (828) 253-1188
FAX (828) 253-8082   e-mail: helpinghomes@nahhh.org
www.nahhh.org

Makes referrals to free or low-cost housing for families receiving medical care away from home. Web site includes listing of hospitality houses by region.

National Association of Inpatient Physicians (NAIP)
190 North Independence Mall West
Philadelphia, PA 19106
(800) 843-3360   (215) 351-2784   www.naiponline.org

Professional organization for physicians (hospitalists) who practice inpatient medicine. Membership, physicians, $140.00; residents/fellows, $40.00; affiliates, $140.00; includes newsletter, "The Hospitalist."

National Patient Safety Foundation (NPSF)
515 North State Street, 8th floor
Chicago, IL 60610
(312) 464-4848   FAX (312) 464-4154   e-mail: info@npsf.org
www.npsf.org

This organization strives to improve patient safety through developing a body of knowledge on the subject, applying the knowledge, developing a culture that is receptive to improving safety, and raising public awareness about the issue. Patient safety literature is available on the web site as are links to related sites.

PUBLICATIONS

The Best Hospitals in America
by John W. Wright and Linda Sunshine
Gale Group
27500 Drake Road
Farmington Hills, MI 48331
(800) 877-4253   FAX (800) 414-5043
e-mail: galegroup@galegroup.com www.galegroup.com

This book describes 387 hospitals that conduct clinical research. Selection of hospitals is based on recommendations by physicians and patient satisfaction. Lists specialties, services, and well known physicians. Includes details on admission policies and room charges. $65.00

Equal Partners: A Physician's Call for a New Spirit of Medicine
by Jody Heymann
Little, Brown and Company, Boston, MA

In this book, a physician whose experiences with severe brain seizures changed her perception of medical care discusses her experiences in the hospital as well as her suggestions for a better form of medicine. Out of print

Hospital Smarts
by Theodore Tyberg and Kenneth Rothaus
Hearst Books, William Morrow and Company

Written by two physicians, this book provides a typical chronology of events that occur when an individual learns that he or she needs to be hospitalized. Includes a number of sample forms that a hospitalized patient will encounter, including DNR (do not resuscitate) documents and health care proxy statements. Out of print.

How to Get Out of the Hospital Alive
by Sheldon Blau and Elaine Fantle Shimberg
Simon and Schuster
100 Front Street
Riverside, NJ 08075
(888) 866-6631   FAX (800) 943-9831   www.simonsays.com

This book discusses the hazards of hospitalization and suggests how patients can advocate for themselves to avoid infection, drug errors, and surgical mistakes. Includes information on diagnostic procedures, medical orders, and patients' rights. $21.95 plus $4.98 shipping and handling

<u>Procedures in U.S. Hospitals, 1997</u>
Agency for Healthcare Research and Quality (AHRQ)
by Anne Elixhauser et al.
Publications Clearinghouse
PO Box 8547
Silver Spring, MD 20907-8547
(800) 358-9295   (888) 586-6340 (TT)   e-mail: info@ahrq.org
www.ahrq.gov

This "Fact Book" reports on the findings from a nationwide sample of inpatient stays. It discusses the most common procedures and who gets them (by age and gender), who pays for the procedures, and mortality rates for procedures at different types of facilities. Free. Also available on the web site.

<u>The Rights of Patients</u>
by George J. Annas
Simon and Schuster
100 Front Street
Riverside, NJ 08075
(888) 866-6631   FAX (800) 943-9831   www.simonsays.com

This book uses a question and answer format to discuss topics such as informed consent, privacy and confidentiality, medical malpractice, and the patient rights movement. $10.95 plus $4.98 shipping and handling

<u>Take Charge of Your Hospital Stay</u>
by Karen Keating McCann
Insight Books

This book provides information about the bureaucratic procedures that take place during a hospital stay and how to deal with them. It also discusses how to obtain information from your physician. Out of print

<u>Take This Book to the Hospital with You</u>
by Charles B. Inlander and Ed Weiner
People's Medical Society
462 Walnut Street
Allentown, PA 18102
(800) 624-8773   FAX (610) 770-0607   www.peoplesmed.org

This book provides information individuals need before, during, and after hospitalization. Includes descriptions of patients' rights and forms for personal recordkeeping of tests and medications, blood pressure and temperature, pain, and interactions with hospital personnel. Members, $11.25; nonmembers, $14.95; plus $4.00 shipping and handling.

To Err is Human: Building a Safer Health System
by Janet Corrigan, Linda Kohn, and Molla Donaldson
National Academy Press
2101 Constitution Avenue, NW
Lockbox 285
Washington, DC 20055
(888) 624-8373   (202) 334-3313   FAX (202) 334-2451
e-mail: zjones@nas.edu   www.nap.edu

This book presents statistics regarding medical errors, an explanation of the forces that contribute to medical errors, as well as suggestions for how patients entering hospitals can influence the care they receive. $34.95 plus $4.50 shipping and handling. Orders placed on the web site receive a discount.

20 Tips To Help Prevent Medical Errors
Agency for Healthcare Research and Quality Publications Clearinghouse
PO Box 8547
Silver Spring, MD 20907-8547
(800) 358-9295   (888) 586-6340 (TT)   e-mail: info@ahrq.gov
www.ahrq.gov

This brochure provides tips for preventing common health care errors. Free

Chapter 5

MEDICAL BENEFITS AND LEGAL RIGHTS

Over the years, the federal government has passed many laws to protect the rights of medical consumers and to establish programs that provide medical benefits. Although most medical consumers are aware of major programs, such as Medicare, there are many specific aspects of these federal programs, including appeals processes, and many nuances of the laws that are not widely known. In order to make wise medical decisions, consumers must know where to turn to obtain information about the laws that affect the health care that they receive. The following sections of this chapter cover major legislation and programs and where to find additional information pertinent to specific situations. Free insurance counseling programs are available through state insurance departments and agencies on aging.

FEDERAL LAWS THAT PROVIDE SPECIFIC MEDICAL RIGHTS

The *Consolidated Omnibus Budget Reconciliation Act of 1985* (P.L. 99-272), more commonly known as COBRA, provides group health insurance continuation to individuals whose work or family status changes due to unemployment, divorce, or a spouse's death or retirement. COBRA requires that employers of 20 or more workers, including local and state governments, provide employees and their families with the option of continuing their group health insurance coverage for 18 months (longer under certain circumstances). This protection was later extended to federal employees and their families. Under COBRA, the individual must pay the entire monthly premium (both the employee and employer portions) and may be charged an administrative fee.

The *Health Insurance Portability and Accountability Act of 1996* (P.L. 104-191), also known as the Kennedy-Kassebaum law or HIPAA, protects individuals from being denied health insurance due to a pre-existing medical condition when they move from one job to another or if they become unemployed. "Portability" means that once individuals have been covered by health insurance, they are credited with having medical coverage when they enter a new plan. Group health plans, health insurance plans such as HMOs, Medicare, Medicaid, military health plans, Indian Health Service medical care, and public, state or federal health benefits are considered creditable coverage (Fuch et al.: 1997). Coverage of a pre-existing medical condition may not be limited for more than 12 months for individuals who enroll in the health plan as soon as they are eligible (18 months for those who delay enrollment). Although the Act creates federal standards, the states have considerable flexibility in their requirements for insurers. The Departments of Treasury, Health and Human Services, and Labor are responsible for enforcing the provisions of the Act.

Protecting the confidentiality of medical records has received some interest in Congress. Bills have been introduced to prohibit discrimination on the basis of genetic information in areas such as employment and insurance. The *Health Insurance Portability and Accountability Act of 1996* also required the Department of Health and Human Services to develop regulations to protect the privacy of individuals' medical records. The regulations went into effect on April 14, 2001. They give consumers the right to see and copy their own medical records and require that consumers provide informed consent before their health information is provided to third parties. Health care plans and providers must provide consumers with a written notice of how they will use the consumers' medical information. Special provisions apply to mental health records. For more detailed information on these regulations, contact the Office for Civil Rights of the Department of Health and Human Services (HHS).

The *Hill-Burton Uncompensated Services Program* requires that certain hospitals and other health facilities that have received federal funds for construction or modernization provide free or low cost health care to individuals whose income falls within poverty income guidelines. Physicians' fees and private pharmacy fees are not covered. A list of Hill-Burton facilities in specific areas is available on request from the Hill-Burton Uncompensated Services Hotline (see "ORGANIZATIONS" section below).

The federal government provides Medicare, Medicaid, and health insurance counseling for Medicare beneficiaries. Your state's department of insurance or state or local department on aging can refer you to these programs.

The *Family and Medical Leave Act of 1993* (P.L. 103-3) requires employers with 50 or more employees at a worksite or within 75 miles of a worksite to permit eligible employees 12 workweeks of unpaid leave during a 12 month period in order to care for themselves, a spouse, son or daughter, or parent who has a serious health condition. During this period of leave, the employer must continue to provide group health benefits for the employee under the same conditions as the employee would have received while working. Upon return from leave, the employee must be restored to the same position he or she had prior to the leave or to a position with equivalent pay, benefits, and conditions of employment. Special regulations apply to employees of school systems and private schools and employees of the federal civil service.

In 1997, Congress passed the *Children's Health Insurance Program* (P.L. 105-33), as part of the Balanced Budget Act of 1997 (CHIP) to make available funds for states to provide insurance for uninsured children of low income, working parents. States have the option of expanding their Medicaid plan or developing a new children's health insurance plan. States are required to submit a plan for approval to the Secretary of Health and Human Services; the law sets standards for what the coverage must include. Eligibility requirements for the program are an income level 200 percent of the poverty level or 50 percentage points above the Medicaid eligibility limit; and children must not be eligible for Medicaid or other health insurance coverage. States must continue Medicaid eligibility for children who would have lost SSI benefits because of the change in the definition of childhood disability under the Personal Responsibility and Work Opportunity Act of 1996.

At the time this book went to press, Congress was debating a "Patients' Bill of Rights," legislation that would increase the rights of patients who obtain their health care from health maintenance organizations (HMOs). Under debate were issues such as whether a cap should be imposed on the awards patients could receive as a result of litigation and, if so, how much it would be and whether the litigation should take place in state or federal courts.

The medical and social service benefits available from organizations receiving federal assistance are guaranteed by federal laws and protected by the Office for Civil Rights of the Department of Health and Human Services (HHS). When an individual feels that his or her rights have been violated, a complaint should be filed with the regional office of HHS (see "ORGANIZATIONS" section below).

FEDERAL HEALTH INSURANCE AND BENEFITS

Medicare is a federal health insurance program for individuals age 65 and older who are eligible for Social Security or Railroad Retirement benefits, those of any age with permanent kidney failure, and some people with disabilities. It is available to individuals regardless of their income or assets. Over 39 million Americans are covered by Medicare (Health Care Financing Administration: 2000). The Social Security Administration is responsible for enrolling Medicare beneficiaries and collecting Medicare premiums. At various times, Congress has considered changes to the Medicare program, such as raising the age for eligibility, instituting income restrictions, and allowing younger people to purchase Medicare insurance.

Medicare has two parts, hospital insurance and medical insurance. Medicare Part A covers inpatient hospital or skilled nursing facility care or care provided by a home health agency or hospice. A portion of Social Security payroll withholding taxes paid by employers and employees and self-employment taxes paid by self-employed persons finances Medicare Part A. If an individual is 65 and a citizen or permanent resident of the United States, and the individual or his or her spouse has worked at least 10 years and made payroll contributions to Medicare, no premium is charged for Medicare Part A. There are, however, deductibles, amounts which the insured must pay before benefits are paid by the insurer, and co-payments, the portion the insured must pay, expressed as either a dollar amount or a percentage. In 2001, for example, under Medicare Part A, before Medicare pays the full cost of the first to 60th day of hospitalization, there is a $792.00 deductible per benefit period. For the 61st to the 90th day of hospitalization, there is a co-insurance of $198.00 a day; for days 91 to 150, $396.00 a day; for all additional days, Medicare pays nothing.

Part B, medical insurance, covers physician bills, outpatient hospital care, and medical services not covered by Part A. It is paid for by a monthly premium which varies with the type of insurance purchased and is often deducted from the individual's Social Security check. After the insured pays a $100.00 annual deductible for Part B, Medicare pays 80% of approved amounts billed for physician and surgical services, medical supplies, diagnostic tests, durable medical equipment, etc. Individuals with low incomes may qualify for a program in which their state pays Medicare premiums and may cover deductibles and co-insurance payments.

Most people purchase *Medicare supplement policies*, often called Medigap policies, to help pay for the gaps in Medicare coverage. Although all Medigap policies must include certain basic benefits, the federal government has mandated ten standardized Medicare supplemental plans. These plans may pay either Part A deductibles, Part A and B deductibles, skilled nursing co-insurance, basic drug expenses, and/or at-home recovery expenses.

Medicaid is a joint federal/state health insurance plan for individuals who are considered financially needy (i.e., recipients of financial benefits from government assistance programs, such as Supplemental Security Income). While federal law requires that each state cover hospital services, skilled nursing facility services, physician and home health care services, and diagnostic and screening services, states have great discretion in other areas.

The federal government provides health and medical services for Alaskan natives and Indians through the Indian Health Service (IHS). Individuals must be enrolled in a recognized tribe or must be able to prove that they are direct descendants of a recognized tribe and must live in the Indian Health Service area. Direct care is provided at IHS clinics, through contract care by referral, or through urban programs with special eligibility criteria. For more information, contact the Indian Health Service at (301) 443-3593 or check a local telephone directory under U.S. Government, "Health and Human Services."

OTHER RESOURCES FOR FINANCIAL ASSISTANCE WITH MEDICAL EXPENSES

You should not overlook private sources for assistance in paying medical expenses. For example, the Pharmaceutical Research and Manufacturers Association (PHRMA) publishes a list of members that offer certain drugs at low or no cost to uninsured or underinsured patients upon submission of a request from a physician. The National Organization for Rare Disorders (NORD) sponsors a Medication Assistance Program and Medical Equipment Exchange for its members.

Within certain guidelines, if you itemize deductions on your income tax return, you may include the costs of meals, lodging, and transportation related to medical care. The National Association of Hospital Hospitality Houses makes referrals to inexpensive lodging for the families of patients who travel long distances for treatment. The Mercy Medical Airlift and other similar organizations provide free air transportation for individuals with medical and financial needs. (See "ORGANIZATIONS" and "PUBLICATIONS AND TAPES" sections below.)

ADVANCE DIRECTIVES

Despite careful investigation and preparation for making wise medical decisions, what will happen if you cannot make your health care wishes known, due to illness or disability? It is important to think about who you want to make decisions for you and to discuss your decisions with family members and your physicians. Do not wait for your physicians to bring up this subject; many physicians think that their patients should initiate the discussion. They are hesitant to talk about discontinuing or withholding treatment. Since accidents and unanticipated illnesses can occur at any time, elders are not the only individuals who should make their health care wishes known.

The *Patient Self-Determination Act of 1990* requires nursing homes, hospices, hospitals, managed care groups, and home health care services to inform service recipients in writing of their rights under state law to have advance directives and to accept or refuse medical care. Since compliance with the Act is an amendment to the Medicare and Medicaid sections of the Social Security Act, some observers have expressed concern about the ethics of linking advance directives with cost containment initiatives (La Puma et al.: 1991). They fear that institutions reimbursed by Medicare, Medicaid, or other plans may try to influence patients' advance directives in areas such as life-sustaining procedures in order to save money on patient care.

The term "advance directive" is used to describe a variety of legal documents including the health care proxy, living will, durable power of attorney, and medical directive. Each state has legal requirements that may affect your decisions. Every state and the District of Columbia have enacted statutes recognizing advance directives (Sabatino: 1994), but the statutes vary in language, restrictions, and procedures. Although generic advance directive forms are available, forms specific to your state are available from local hospitals, bar associations, state or local offices on aging, or state or local medical or hospital associations. For a nominal fee, Partnership for Caring, a national organization (see "ORGANIZATIONS" section below), will provide forms that meet your state's legal requirements. Individuals who join the organization receive information about changes in their own state's laws that may affect their advance directives.

A *living will* is used to tell your doctors and family members of your choices about medical treatment if you are terminally ill, unconscious, or unable to communicate. With a *health care power of attorney*, you designate another person to be your health care agent, in order to make decisions for you when you are unable to make them yourself. It is wise to name a principal health care agent as well as an alternate. In some states, the health care agent is called a health care proxy. Advance directives may be changed at any time. They should be witnessed by disinterested parties and placed in your medical records. It is wise to carry a card in your wallet indicating the identity of your health care agent and where your advance directive may be found. Your advance directive should be part of your hospital record when you are admitted for treatment, and a copy should be sent with you if you are transferred from one facility to another, as from an acute care hospital to a rehabilitation center or from a nursing home to a hospital.

There are many issues to consider when preparing a living will or a health care power of attorney. You should discuss these issues with your primary care physician, your family, and your designated agents. For example:

- How do you feel about receiving treatments such as cardiopulmonary resuscitation (CPR), mechanical respiration, artificial feeding, kidney dialysis, blood transfusions, invasive diagnostic tests, major or minor surgery, chemotherapy, or antibiotics if you are in a coma with no chance of recovery?
- Would you feel differently if you were in a coma but had a small chance of regaining consciousness?
- Would you choose to be treated for a life-threatening but reversible illness if you already had an incurable condition that would ultimately lead to death?
- How do you feel about being an organ donor?
- How important is independence to you?

In order to make decisions on your behalf, your health care proxy should be aware of your beliefs and wishes. In preparing a living will, you may wish to include specific statements regarding continuation of life-sustaining procedures, such as resuscitation or artificial nutrition and hydration. You may wish to place time constraints on these decisions. For instance, you may want to state a limit to the number of days you remain in an irreversible vegetative state before life-sustaining procedures are discontinued. You may also use this document to state your preferences about nursing home placement or dying at home. A study of individuals who had prepared advance directives showed that their treatment choices remained the same one to two years after they made these decisions (Emanuel et al.: 1994); nonetheless, you should review your advance directives at regular intervals to be certain that you still want the same stipulations.

Even if you are certain that you have completed the advance directives so that they meet the legal requirements of your state, they are useless unless members of your family, your health agent, and your physicians are aware of them and of your wishes regarding medical treatment. A study (Virmani et al.: 1994) found that physicians were frequently unaware of their patients' advance directives and that the majority of patients studied had not discussed their treatment wishes with their physicians. Another study (Teno et al.: 1997) found that not only do the few patients who have written advance directives fail to inform their physicians about them, but most of the advance directives are too vague for physicians to understand what the patients want done in specific situations. Yet another study found that physicians' own personal preferences influenced their perceptions of patients' preferences on interventions such as cardiopulmonary resuscitation, tube feeding, and artificial hydration (Schneiderman et al.: 1993).

The importance of having clear and specific directives is apparent in emergency situations. For example, when emergency medical teams are called in when a patient has no heartbeat, they are required to attempt to resuscitate the patients unless they have legal proof of "do not resuscitate" orders. In many cases, this evidence is not available at the time they are called to help.

In order to make clear advance directives that your health agent and physicians are able to follow, read as much as possible on the topic. Collect the forms that are legally binding in your state. Discuss your wishes with your family, significant others, and primary care physician. Then consult an attorney who specializes in health issues to ensure that your documents are clear and will stand up under legal scrutiny.

References

Emanuel, L.L. et al.
1994 "Advance Directives: Stability of Patients' Treatment Choices" <u>Archives of Internal Medicine</u> 154:(January):209-217
Fuch, Beth C. et al.
1997 <u>The Health Insurance Portability and Accountability Act of 1996: Guidance</u> Washington DC: Library of Congress, Congressional Research Service
Health Care Financing Administration
2000 <u>Medicare 2000: 35 Years of Improving Americans' Health and Security</u> Baltimore, MD: Health Care Financing Administration
La Puma, John et al.
1991 "Advance Directives on Admission" <u>JAMA</u> 256:3(July 17):402-405
Sabatino, Charles P.
1994 "Ten Legal Myths About Advance Medical Directives" <u>Clearinghouse Review</u> 28:6(October):653-657

Schneiderman, L.J., R.M. Kaplan, and R.A. Pearlman

1993   "Do Physicians' Own Preferences for Life-Sustaining Treatment Influence Their Perceptions of Patients' Preferences?" Journal of Clinical Ethics 4(1):18-33

Teno, Joan et al.

1997   "Do Advance Directives Provide Instructions that Direct Care?" Journal of the American Geriatrics Society 45:500-507

Virmani, J., L.J. Schneiderman, and R.M. Kaplan

1994   "Relationship of Advance Directives to Physician-Patient Communication" Archives of Internal Medicine 154(April):909-913

ORGANIZATIONS

American Bar Association Commission on Legal Problems of the Elderly
740 15th Street, NW
Washington, DC 20005
(202) 662-8690   FAX (202) 662-8698
e-mail: abaelderly@abanet.org   www.abanet.org/elderly

Advocates on behalf of elders in areas such as health care decision-making, housing, elder abuse, public benefits, age discrimination, and guardianship. Free publications list.

BenefitsCheckup.org
National Council on Aging

This interactive web site has the user enter information about health conditions, disabilities, income, and assets (entries are held in private) and responds with a list of benefits the user is eligible for and the agencies to contact in the user's local area.

Center for Medicare Advocacy
PO Box 350
Willimantic, CT 06226
(800) 262-4414   (860) 456-7790
www.medicareadvocacy.org

This center, staffed by attorneys who specialize in Medicare issues, provides legal assistance and representation as well as self-help materials. Represents clients who want to appeal Medicare decisions, especially the denial of home health care. Services are free to Connecticut residents and provided for a fee to others. Free publications list.

Centers for Medicare and Medicaid Services (CMS)
formerly Health Care Financing Administration (HCFA)
7500 Security Boulevard
Baltimore, MD 21244
(800) 633-4227   (410) 786-3000   www.hcfa.gov
www.medicare.gov

CMS is the federal agency that administers Medicare and Medicaid. Current Medicare regulations are available on the web site, as are many publications, including those about health care plans and the appeals process for federal benefits.

Federal Trade Commission (FTC)
600 Pennsylvania Avenue, NW
Washington, DC 20580
(877) 382-4357   (202) 326-4357   www.ftc.gov

This federal agency is mandated to protect consumers against unfair, deceptive, or fraudulent practices, including advertising, marketing, and sales of over-the-counter drugs, health care goods, and services. Ten regional offices. Free publications list. Publications are also available on the web site.

Food and Drug Administration (FDA)
Office of Consumer Affairs
5600 Fishers Lane
Rockville, MD 20857
(888) 463-6332   (301) 827-4420   FAX (301) 443-9767
e-mail: execsec@oc.fda.gov   www.fda.gov

This federal agency regulates items shipped in interstate commerce such as food, drugs, medical devices, electronic products (laser products, ultrasonic therapy equipment, radiation devices), biologics, and veterinary products. Publishes newsletter, "FDA Consumer," $13.50 (six issues); free on FDA's web site, which includes back issues and index. To report fraudulent claims appearing on the Internet, send e-mail: otcfraud@cder.fda.gov

Health Insurance Association of America (HIAA)
1201 F Street, NW, Suite 500
Washington, DC 20004
(800) 879-4422   (202) 824-1600   FAX (202) 824-1722
www.hiaa.org

Trade association of insurers and managed care companies. Publishes "The Consumer Guide to Long-Term Care Insurance;" single copy, free. Also available on the web site.

Health Privacy Project of Georgetown University
2233 Wisconsin Avenue, NW, Suite 525
Washington, DC 20007
(202) 687-0880   FAX (202) 784-1265   www.healthprivacy.org

This organization provides resources on public policies regarding health privacy, especially federal protections mandated by the federal government.

Hill-Burton Uncompensated Services Program Hotline
(800) 638-0742   In Maryland, (800) 492-0359
www.hrsa.dhhs.gov/osp

This hotline provides information on the Hill-Burton program and a brochure, "Free Hospital Care," that describes the program and instructions on filing an application. Free

Internal Revenue Service (IRS)
(800) 829-1040   (800) 829-4059 (TT)
www.irs.ustreas.gov

The IRS provides technical assistance about tax credits and deductions related to medical expenses and accommodations for disabilities. To receive Publication 502, "Medical and Dental Expenses," Publication 554, "Older Americans' Tax Guide," Publication 501, "Exemptions, Standard Deduction, and Filing Information;" Publication 907, "Tax Highlights for Persons with Disabilities;" and Publication 524, "Credit for the Elderly or the Disabled," call (800) 829-3676; (800) 829-4059 (TT). These publications are also available on the web site.

Medicare Health Plan Compare
www.hcfa.gov   www.medicare.gov

Provides access to information about Medicare managed care plans so that consumers may compare costs, premiums, and the types of services provided.

Medicare Hotline
(800) 633-4227

This toll-free hotline, sponsored by the Centers for Medicare and Medicaid Services (CMS) (formerly HCFA, Health Care Financing Administration), provides information for Medicare beneficiaries and their families including general information, claims, publications, and information on Medicare coverage. Information is available in English and Spanish.

Mercy Medical Airlift
9998 Wakefield Drive, Suite 110
Manassas, VA 20110
(800) 296-1191, extension 23   (703) 296-1191, extension 23
FAX (703) 257-1642   e-mail: mercymedical@erols.com
National Patient Air Transport Helpline: (800) 296-1217   www.npath.org

Provides charitable air transportation for individuals with medical and financial needs.

National Association of Hospital Hospitality Houses (NAHHH)
PO Box 18087
Asheville, NC 28814-0087
(800) 542-9730   (828) 253-1188
FAX (828) 253-8082   e-mail: helpinghomes@nahhh.orgwww.nahhh.org

Makes referrals to free or low-cost housing for families receiving medical care away from home. Web site includes listing of hospitality houses by region.

National Committee for Quality Assurance (NCQA)
2000 L Street, NW, Suite 500
Washington, DC 20036
(888) 275-7585   (202) 955-3500
FAX (202) 955-3599   www.ncqa.org

An organization that evaluates and accredits health care plans so that consumers may have the information to make informed decisions about choosing a health care plan. NCQA will tell consumers whether a specific plan is accredited and provide a summary of the evaluation report. Summaries also appear on the NCQA web site.

National Consumers League (NCL)
1701 K Street, NW, Suite 1200
Washington, DC 20006
(202) 835-3323   FAX (202) 835-0747   www.nclnet.org

This national consumer organization advocates for access to affordable health care and truth in labeling of food, drugs, and cosmetics. Publishes brochures on health care and food and drug safety. Membership, $20.00, includes newsletter "NCL Bulletin," legislative updates, and discounts on publications and conferences. Also operates the National Fraud Information Center; (800) 876-7060; www.fraud.org

National Organization for Rare Disorders (NORD)
100 Rt. 37, PO Box 8923
New Fairfield, CT 06812-8923
(800) 999-6673   (203) 746-6518   (203) 746-6927 (TT)
FAX (203) 746-6481   e-mail: orphan@rarediseases.org
www.rarediseases.org

This federation of voluntary health organizations that serves individuals with rare or "orphan" diseases advocates for public policy issues such as privacy of medical records, orphan drug tax credits, and children's health insurance. Offers Medical Equipment Exchange on web site to link buyers and sellers of used medical equipment and a Medication Assistance Program. Maintains a confidential patient networking program for individuals and family members who have been diagnosed with a rare disorder. Membership, $30.00. Reprints of articles on rare diseases available from the NORD Rare Disease Database for $7.50 per copy; abstracts available free on web site. Publishes quarterly newsletter, "Orphan Disease Update." Free

Nolo Law for All
Nolo Press
950 Parker Street
Berkeley, CA 94710
(800) 992-6656   FAX (800) 645-0895   e-mail: cs@nolo.com
www.nolo.com

This online service provides information on legal topics, updates legislation and court decisions, and features articles from "Nolo News." Free publications catalogue.

Office for Civil Rights, Department of Health and Human Services
200 Independence Avenue, SW
Washington, DC 20201
(877) 696-6775   (202) 619-0700   (202) 863-0101 (TT)
FAX (202) 619-3818   www.hhs.gov

Responsible for enforcing laws and regulations that protect the rights of individuals seeking medical and social services in institutions that receive federal financial assistance. Individuals who feel their rights have been violated may file a complaint with one of the ten regional offices located throughout the country. Calling (800) 368-1019 connects you with the regional office closed to you. A special phone number has been established for the office that enforces the health privacy regulations, (866) 827-7748 or e-mail to ocrprivacy@os.dhhs.gov

Partnership for Caring
PO Box 97290
Washington, DC 20077-7205
(800) 989-9455   (202) 296-8071
FAX (202) 296-8352   e-mail: pfc@partnershipforcaring.org
www.partnershipforcaring.org

Provides advance directive forms (living will and medical power of attorney) tailored to individual state legal requirements; $5.00 per set. Advance directive forms may be downloaded from web site, free. Membership, $35.00, includes quarterly newsletter, "Choices."

Privacy Rights Clearinghouse
1717 Kettner Avenue, Suite 105
San Diego, CA 92101
(619) 298-3396   FAX (619) 298-5681
e-mail: prc@privacyrights.org   www.privacyrights.org

This organization provides information about how consumers can protect their medical and financial information as well as information about the latest laws regarding privacy. Many fact sheets are available on the web site. Free

Social Security Administration
6401 Security Boulevard
Baltimore, MD 21235
(800) 772-1213   (800) 325-0778 (TT)   www.ssa.gov

To obtain a copy of a "Request for Earnings and Benefit Estimate Statement," call the number above. To apply for Social Security benefits based on disability, call to set up an appointment with a Social Security representative, or visit the local Social Security office. Publishes monthly "eNews" online newsletter, free.

Thomas
Library of Congress
thomas.loc.gov

This online service provides a database of recent laws and pending legislation, as well as information about the committees of Congress and the text of the "Congressional Record." Searches for legislation and laws may be done by topic or public law number. Since changes are expected in Social Security, Medicare, Medicaid, and other government programs, this database is a good resource for the status of pending legislation.

PUBLICATIONS AND TAPES

The ABA Legal Guide for Older Americans
American Bar Association Commission on Legal Problems of the Elderly
740 15th Street, NW
Washington, DC 20005
(202) 662-8690   FAX (202) 662-8698
e-mail: abaelderly@abanet.org   www.abanet.org/elderly

This guide provides information on topics such as health care, health and long term care insurance, advance directives, Medicare, Medicaid, Medigap, and housing. $13.00

Advance Directives and the Elderly: Making Decisions About Treatment Limitations
Video Press
University of Maryland School of Medicine
100 North Greene Street, Suite 300
Baltimore, MD 21201
(800) 328-7450   (410) 706-5497   FAX (410) 706-8471
www.videopress.org

In this videotape, three nursing home residents discuss with their physician their wishes regarding cardiopulmonary resuscitation, artificial feeding, and the use of antibiotics. 20 minutes. Purchase, $150.00; two week rental, $75.00.

Advance Directives: CPR in Nursing Homes
Video Press
University of Maryland School of Medicine
100 North Greene Street, Suite 300
Baltimore, MD 21201
(800) 328-7450   (410) 706-5497   FAX (410) 706-8471
www.videopress.org

In this videotape, a physician, a nursing home resident, and the resident's daughter discuss cardiopulmonary resuscitation. Includes basic information and emotional concerns. 19 minutes. Purchase, $150.00; two week rental, $75.00.

Artificial Nutrition and Hydration and End-of-Life Decision Making
Partnership for Caring
PO Box 97290
Washington, DC 20077-7205
(800) 989-9455   (202) 296-8071
FAX (202) 296-8352   e-mail: pfc@partnershipforcaring.org
www.partnershipforcaring.org

This booklet provides information on tube feeding and patient comfort for individuals faced with making these decisions. $5.95

The Consumer's Legal Guide to Today's Health Care
by Stephen L. Isaacs and Ava C. Schwartz
Houghton Mifflin Company, Boston, MA

This book describes patients' legal rights regarding treatment options, insurance (including Medicare and medical supplemental insurance), long term care, the right to die, and the need for a lawyer. Out of print

Directory of Legal Aid and Defender Offices
National Legal Aid and Defender Association
1625 K Street, NW, 8th floor
Washington, DC 20006
(202) 452-0620   FAX (202) 872-1031   www.nlads.org

A directory of legal aid offices throughout the U.S. Includes chapters on disability protection/advocacy, health law, and senior citizens. Updated biennially. $70.00

Directory of Prescription Drug Patient Assistance Programs
Pharmaceutical Research and Manufacturers Association (PHRMA)
1100 15th Street, NW
Washington, DC 20005
(800) 762-4636   (202) 835-3400   www.phrma.org

A list of members that offer certain drugs at low or no cost to uninsured or underinsured patients. Most programs require that a physician make the request. Free

Federal Benefits for Veterans and Dependents
(800) 827-1000   www.va.gov

This booklet describes the benefits available under federal laws. Available from the Department of Veterans Affairs or any VA regional office. Free

Federal Register
New Orders, Superintendent of Documents
PO Box 371954
Pittsburgh, PA 15250-7954
(866) 512-1800   (202) 512-1530
FAX (202) 512-2250   e-mail: gpoaccess@gpo.gov
www.access.gpo.gov/su_docs/aces/aces140.html

A federal publication printed every weekday with notices of all regulations and legal notices issued by federal agencies. Domestic subscriptions, $764.00 annually for second class mailing of paper format; $264.00 annually for microfiche. Access to the Federal Register is available through the Internet at the address listed above at no charge.

Five Wishes
Aging with Dignity
PO Box 1661
Tallahassee, FL 32302
(888) 594-7437   (850) 681-2010   FAX (850) 681-2481
e-mail: fivewishes@agingwithdignity.org
www.agingwithdignity.org

A living will that covers an individual's medical, personal, emotional, and spiritual needs and is legally valid in 35 states. $5.00. The "Five Wishes Video" may be used to encourage discussion among family members. 25 minutes. $19.95 plus $7.00 shipping and handling. "Next Steps Guide" is a booklet that offers suggestions on talking with loved ones and doctors about "Five Wishes." $5.00.

Guide to Using the Family and Medical Leave Act: Questions and Answers
National Partnership for Women and Families
1875 Connecticut Avenue, NW, Suite 710
Washington, DC 20009
(202) 986-2600   FAX (202) 986-2539
www.nationalpartnership.org

This booklet answers the most frequently asked questions about the law. Available in English and Spanish. Free. Also available on the web site.

Health and Financial Decisions: Legal Tools for Preserving Personal Autonomy
American Bar Association Commission on Legal Problems of the Elderly
740 15th Street, NW
Washington, DC 20005
(202) 662-8690   FAX (202) 662-8698
e-mail: abaelderly@abanet.org   www.abanet.org/elderly

This brochure provides information on advance directives, powers of attorney, trusts, and living wills. $1.00

Health Benefits Under the Consolidated Omnibus Budget Reconciliation Act (COBRA)
U.S. Department of Labor
Pension and Welfare Benefits Administration
Division of Technical Assistance and Inquiries
200 Constitution Avenue, NW, Room N5656
Washington, DC 20210
(800) 998-7542 (Publications Order Line)   (202) 219-8921
(800) 501-3911 (TT)   www.dol.gov/dol/pwba

This booklet describes the requirements of this program which enables former employees in the private sector, state and local governments to continue health coverage at group rates. Free. Also available on the web site.

Health Insurance: How To Get It, Keep It, or Improve What You've Got
by Robert Enteen
Demos Vermande
386 Park Avenue South, Suite 201
New York, NY 10016
(800) 532-8663   (212) 683-0072   FAX (212) 683-0118
e-mail: info@demospub.com   www.demosmedpub.com

This book helps medical consumers locate and evaluate health insurance plans. Also discusses health insurance options including managed care and long term care insurance. $29.95 plus $4.00 shipping and handling. Orders placed on the web site receive a 15% discount.

Living Wills
Films for the Humanities and Sciences
PO Box 2053
Princeton, NJ 08543
(800) 257-5126   FAX (609) 275-3767
e-mail: custserv@films.com   www.films.com

In this videotape, patients, families, and physicians discuss the preparation of advance directives. 30 minutes. Purchase, $89.95; rental, $75.00; plus 6% shipping and handling

The Medical Marketplace
Aquarius Health Care Videos
5 Powderhouse Lane
PO Box 1159
Sherborn, MA 01770
(888) 440-2963   (508) 651-2963   FAX (508) 650-4216
e-mail: ordering@aquariusproductions.com
www.aquariusproductions.com

This videotape discusses the relationship between patients and health care providers. Provides guidelines assessing medical information and for evaluating health care providers. 28 minutes. Purchase, $99.00; one day rental, $50.00; one week rental, $100.00; plus $10.00 shipping and handling

Medicare & You
Centers for Medicare and Medicaid Services (CMS)
formerly Health Care Financing Administration (HCFA)
7500 Security Boulevard
Baltimore, MD 21244
(800) 633-4227   (410) 786-3000   www.hcfa.gov
www.medicare.gov

This booklet provides basic information about Medicare including eligibility, enrollment, coverage, and options. Free. Available in English and Spanish in print and audiocassette; in English in large print and braille. Also available on the web site.

Medicare Appeals and Grievances
Centers for Medicare and Medicaid Services (CMS)
formerly Health Care Financing Administration (HCFA)
7500 Security Boulevard
Baltimore, MD 21244
(800) 633-4227   (410) 786-3000   www.hcfa.gov
www.medicare.gov

This publication provides information on how to appeal denials of coverage. Also available on the web site.

Planning for Uncertainty: A Guide to Living Wills and Other Advance Directives for Health Care
by David John Doukas and William Reichel
Johns Hopkins University Press
PO Box 50370
Baltimore, MD 21211-4370
(800) 537-5487   FAX (410) 516-6998   www.press.jhu.edu/press

This book discusses various advance directives such as living wills and durable power of attorney. Includes a values history that individuals may wish to consider as they document their personal medical choices. $16.95

Selecting Medicare Supplemental Insurance
American Association of Retired Persons (AARP)
601 E Street, NW
Washington, DC 20049
(800) 424-3410   (202) 434-2277   www.aarp.org

This booklet describes the gaps in Medicare coverage and makes suggestions for purchasing Medigap insurance. Free

A Shopper's Guide to Long-Term Care Insurance
National Association of Insurance Commissioners (NAIC)
2301 McGee, Suite 80
Kansas City, MO 64108
(816) 842-3600   FAX (816) 783-8175   e-mail: pubdist@naic.org
www.naic.org

This booklet provides an overview of long term care insurance, describing the types of policies available, benefits, eligibility requirements, and costs. Includes lists of state insurance departments, agencies on aging, and insurance counseling programs. Two worksheets help consumers evaluate the availability and costs of local long term care and compare policies. $.60

2000 Guide to Health Insurance for People with Medicare
National Association of Insurance Commissioners (NAIC)
2301 McGee, Suite 80
Kansas City, MO 64108
(816) 842-3600   FAX (816) 783-8175   e-mail: pubdist@naic.org
www.naic.org

This booklet provides guidance for purchase of health insurance supplements and describes 10 standardized plans. Single copy, $.80. Also available on the web site.

2001 Guide to Health Insurance for People with Medicare: Choosing a Medigap Policy
Centers for Medicare and Medicaid Services (CMS)
formerly Health Care Financing Administration (HCFA)
7500 Security Boulevard
Baltimore, MD 21244
(800) 633-4227   (410) 786-3000   www.hcfa.gov
www.medicare.gov

This book provides basic information on the two parts of Medicare, what Medicare and medigap policies cover, how much medigap policies cost, and your rights to purchase medigap insurance. Available in large print (English and Spanish), audiocassette (English and Spanish), and braille. Free

WillMaker 8
Nolo Press Self-Help Law Books & Software
950 Parker Street
Berkeley, CA 94710
(800) 992-6656   FAX (800) 645-0895   e-mail: cs@nolo.com
www.nolo.com

This software helps individuals prepare a will as well as a living will and durable power of attorney. Macintosh and Windows versions available. $39.95 plus $5.00 shipping and handling. Orders placed on the web site receive a discount.

Worksheet for Comparing Medicare Health Plans
Centers for Medicare and Medicaid Services (CMS)
formerly Health Care Financing Administration (HCFA)
7500 Security Boulevard
Baltimore, MD 21244
(800) 633-4227   (410) 786-3000   www.hcfa.gov
www.medicare.gov

This booklet provides worksheets that allow space for comparing three Medicare health plans. Suggests questions to ask each plan provider. Also available on the web site.

Your Medical Rights
by Charles B. Inlander and Eugene I. Pavalon
People's Medical Society
462 Walnut Street
Allentown, PA 18102
(800) 624-8773   FAX (610) 770-0607   www.peoplesmed.org

This book describes patients' medical rights, such as disclosure of information, right to privacy, informed consent, and advance directives. It discusses malpractice and filing complaints against practitioners. Includes a doctor information worksheet and individual medical record forms. $14.95 plus $4.00 shipping and handling

Your Medicare Rights
American Association of Retired Persons (AARP)
601 E Street, NW
Washington, DC 20049
(800) 424-3410   (202) 434-2277   www.aarp.org

This booklet describes Medicare rights and outlines the process to appeal denials of care and coverage. Free

Chapter 6

DRUGS

Assuming that drugs approved by the government are safe, many medical consumers take prescription medications without knowing how they work and what side effects they cause. Once a drug has been approved to treat a certain condition, it does not need additional approval to be used for other conditions. In many instances, the prescribed dosage should be related to the individual's medical condition or to body weight. Safety conscious medical consumers should check the warnings and instructions prior to taking drugs that have been prescribed by their physicians.

It is always wise to find out about drugs and their side effects and contraindications, but this is especially important when in the hospital. More than six percent of all hospital patients experience an adverse drug event (Bates et al.: 1999). If surgery is planned, question the physician beforehand to learn about the drugs that will be administered during and after surgery. After surgery, patients are not fully alert and should make prior arrangements with a personal advocate to check the medications and doses that are being administered. Individuals who are receiving chemotherapy for cancer treatment should be especially careful to inquire about the drugs and dosages that will be administered. A case of an overdose prescribed for an experimental drug to treat breast cancer at a prestigious cancer institute in Boston resulted in the death of one woman and serious injury to another. Because the woman who died had been a medical columnist for the <u>Boston Globe</u>, the story received a great deal of publicity. It is likely that incidents such as this occur commonly but do not receive publicity because the individuals involved are not well known.

ADVERSE DRUG EVENTS

Adverse drug events (ADEs) are injuries from medical intervention rather than disease. ADEs are an important consideration when a new drug is submitted to the Food and Drug Administration (FDA) for approval. The clinical trials in which new drugs are studied are limited in scope; they are usually too short, use too small a sample of subjects, study only certain groups, and focus on the drug's effectiveness with a specific disease to anticipate all possible reactions. In 1993, for example, the FDA approved an antiepileptic drug, felbamate (felbatol), for use in reducing partial seizures. A year later, there were reports of nine cases of aplastic anemia, a rare but fatal bone marrow condition, in an estimated 100,000 patients who had taken the drug. As a result, the FDA recommended that physicians discontinue the use of felbamate. The clinical trials conducted on felbamate had not encountered any cases of aplastic anemia (Food and Drug Administration: 1995).

In another example, rezulin (troglitazone) was approved by the FDA for treating type 2 diabetes. Less than a year after it had been on the market, a number of cases of liver damage were attributed to the drug, including some cases that were fatal. In this case, the drug was not immediately taken off the market, but warnings about monitoring liver function were issued to physicians and patients. Eventually, however, the drug was removed from the market.

Drugs tested by the FDA do not undergo long term administration; therefore, the long term effects of new drugs on the market are unknown. When a new drug is prescribed and has no long term track record, medical consumers must weigh the known risks and benefits and the seriousness of the condition being treated; then they must make a decision using all available information.

In addition to causing patients pain and suffering, ADEs account for longer hospital stays and increased hospital costs. Bates (1997) reported that individuals who had had preventable ADEs remained in the hospital more than four and a half days longer than patients who had not had an ADE. A preventable ADE cost $4,685.00 in additional expenses to the hospital. Leape and his colleagues (1995) found that the incidence of ADEs could be decreased if hospitals undertook actions such as standardizing drug orders, upgrading computer systems, and improving communications between physicians and nurses. Bates (1998) found that a physician computer order entry system reduced ADEs by 55%.

Although one might speculate that physicians' notoriously poor handwriting accounts for drug errors or dispensing errors on the part of pharmacists, research shows that ADEs are most frequently made at the drug order or dosage stage and the errors are made by physicians who do not know enough about the drug or the patient for whom it is being prescribed. Organizations such as the Joint Commission on Accreditation of Healthcare Organizations and the American Society of Health-System Pharmacists have devised standards for reporting ADEs, although individual health care professionals do so primarily on a voluntary basis. The FDA's MedWatch (see "ORGANIZATIONS" section below) program was established to encourage professionals to report serious events, i.e., those that are fatal, permanently or significantly disabling, life-threatening, requiring or prolonging hospitalization, or requiring intervention to prevent permanent impairment or damage (Food and Drug Administration: 1996).

Despite the increasing number of safeguards instituted to prevent ADEs, hospital patients must continue to protect themselves by asking, before any injection or pill is administered, "What is this drug? What is it for?" Hospital personnel should always check your identification bracelet to ascertain that you are the intended recipient. The wristband should list your drug allergies. Although you may tire of endless questions about drug allergies asked by all personnel who enter your hospital room, answer them carefully and thoroughly.

Whenever a physician prescribes a new medication, you should ask the following questions:

- What is the name of the medication, both proprietary (brand name) and generic? Can I take a generic form? If not, why not?
- How long has the drug been on the market? How long has it been used for my condition?
- Is the drug available over-the-counter (OTC)? In some cases, the OTC form of a drug may only be available in lower doses and may be more expensive than the same drug in prescription form.
- What is this medication supposed to do for my condition? How does it work?

- Should I avoid driving while I am taking this medicine?
- What happens if I miss a dose?
- Will this medication affect my sleep, or will I feel tired while taking it?
- What are the possible side effects?
- Will cutting the pills in half or crushing them so that swallowing will be easier cause a problem? Some drugs are coated to delay absorption in the body and lose this property if split.
- When should I expect to have relief of my symptoms? Some medicines, such as antibiotics, must be taken for a certain period of time in order to have the desired effect.
- Are there any special instructions for storing this medicine? Should it be refrigerated? Kept in a dry location? Will it lose its effectiveness after some period of time? How often may I renew the prescription?
- Will the drug have deleterious interactions with other drugs I am taking?
- If I have an adverse experience, is it possible to prescribe something else? For example, many people experience gastrointestinal problems when taking the antibiotic erythromycin.

If your physician does not provide the information that you need about a medication, ask your pharmacist. Many pharmacies provide a computer printout with pertinent information about the prescription. Legislation on the state and federal levels requires pharmacists to offer drug counseling to their customers. The Health Care Financing Administration requires that Medicaid recipients receive information including a description of the drug, the dose prescribed, and how long it should be taken. The Physicians' Desk Reference, available in bookstores and libraries, is an excellent resource for learning about drugs, precautions, and adverse reactions.

OVER-THE-COUNTER DRUGS

Over-the-counter (OTC) or nonprescription drugs are those which have been approved by the FDA for use without a physician's prescription. When purchasing these drugs, you have the responsibility for understanding what you are taking and reading the label for instructions. OTC products must be labeled with the following information: the product name; ingredients; what conditions the product is used to treat; usual dosage for adults and for children; warnings, such as possible side effects, when to stop taking the medicine, or when to see your doctor; and an expiration date. If you have questions, ask the pharmacist, call your physician, or look up the drug in the Physicians' Desk Reference for Nonprescription Drugs (see "PUBLICATIONS" section below).

You should tell your physician if you are taking both prescription and nonprescription drugs, since there may be dangerous interactions. Some OTC products should not be taken when you are having certain symptoms. For example, some nasal sprays are contraindicated for people with heart, thyroid, or prostate disease, diabetes, or high blood pressure. Alcohol should be avoided in combination with many OTC products. These warnings appear on OTC labels; however, information changes, so you should read the labels each time you purchase a new supply. If you are pregnant, discuss all medications, prescription and nonprescription, with your physician, since they may not be safe for the fetus. Many medications should also be avoided when breastfeeding.

PAIN CONTROL

The provision of adequate pain control has been problematic for many years among mainstream physicians in the United States. Although protocols for administering pain medication successfully have been developed, many physicians fail to provide adequate pain medication for fear that the patients will become drug addicts. Those physicians who administer appropriate pain control medications are not hesitant to criticize their colleagues for failing to provide adequate pain medication:

> The most common error made by physicians in managing severe
> pain with opioids is to prescribe an inadequate dose. Since many
> patients are reluctant to complain, this practice leads to needless
> suffering. (Fields and Martin: 1994, p. 52)

When administered properly, opioids such as morphine and codeine are highly effective in controlling pain. Individuals who were not previously addicted to drugs will not require drugs after the pain of an illness or surgery has abated. When pain is under control, patients not only feel better, but they may require a shorter hospital stay, have reduced medical expenses, and return to everyday activities sooner. Administered properly, pain medication will not interfere with mental functioning. Compounding the problem of physicians underprescribing pain medication is the failure of nurses to administer the medication that has been prescribed (Honaker: 1995). A large study (Desbiens et al.: 1996) of seriously ill patients in five teaching hospitals found that satisfaction with pain control varied significantly among the hospitals, suggesting that the culture of the hospital regarding pain control makes a difference in how physicians administer pain medication.

One form of pain control that has been developed is called intravenous patient-controlled analgesia (PCA). PCA enables patients to release a narcotic as they need it. Clinicians pre-set the dosages and intervals to prevent overdosing (Walker: 1995). PCA allows patients to self-administer pain relief without calling -- and waiting -- for a nurse. Spinal or epidural administration of pain control medications may avoid side effects such as nausea and vomiting but may induce bladder problems.

Some people think that they should wait as long as possible before taking pain control medication. If they wait longer than the indicated interval, the pain may become worse and the medication may take longer to have its desired effect. If medicines are taken according to the prescribed schedule and they are not effective, the physician should be informed, and he or she should adjust the dosage or frequency or prescribe a different medication.

Cultural attitudes toward pain are often unrecognized by health care personnel. While some cultures believe that expressing feelings of pain is taboo, others sanction free expression of pain. These beliefs may lead health care professionals to overestimate or underestimate an individual's pain tolerance and affect the prescription of pain control medications.

In 1999, the Joint Commission on Accreditation of Healthcare Organizations (JCAHO) (See "ORGANIZATIONS" section below) developed a set of standards for pain management. Beginning in 2001, scores will be calculated for compliance with these standards.

Pain clinics or centers are sources of help for people who experience chronic pain. More than 800 pain clinics or centers in the United States are settings where a multidisciplinary team of health care providers designs an individualized treatment plan for each patient. A variety of treatment modalities is used for each patient, including exercise, diet modification, individual or group psychotherapy, massage, and analgesic medications. The Commission on Accreditation of Rehabilitation Facilities accredits pain programs in the United States, Canada, and Sweden (see "ORGANIZATIONS" section below). For a list of physicians who specialize in pain management, call your local medical society or the American Academy of Pain Medicine (see "ORGANIZATIONS" section below). When considering a pain management program or physician, ask about experience in treating your condition or disability; treatment outcomes, such as return to work or independent living; "graduate" satisfaction; and the average length and cost of treatment. A chronic pain support group may offer practical information and emotional support through the experiences of others (see Chapter 1, "Talking with Other Medical Consumers" section).

Be sure that your wishes about pain control are included in your advance directive (see Chapter 5, "Advance Directives" section). Discuss these concerns with your physician so that you will be aware of the drugs that are available to keep you pain-free and any side effects they may have.

PAIN CONTROL FOR INDIVIDUALS WHO HAVE CANCER

Cancer pain may be caused by the cancer itself or by treatment, such as radiation. Removal of a tumor that is pressing on a nerve, organ, or bone may relieve pain but may result in post-surgical pain. When pain is under control, hospital stays may be shorter, and fewer post-surgical complications may occur. Radiation or chemotherapy may be used to shrink tumors in order to reduce pain but may cause pain themselves. Other non-surgical pain control options include prescription and nonprescription pain relievers; noninvasive methods such as relaxation exercises, imagery, and massage; and anesthetic techniques, such as freezing or epidural infusions that block nerves.

A study found that oncologists are more knowledgeable about pain control than primary care physicians. Neither specialty had ideal behavior when it came to pain control for their patients, but the oncologists were more likely to administer better pain control (Levin et al.: 1998). Recognizing that many cancer patients receive inadequate pain treatment, in 1994 the Agency for Health Care Policy and Research developed guidelines for treating cancer pain. Management of Cancer Pain provides guidelines for assessing and managing pain, using a variety of techniques, including drugs, behavioral strategies, palliative radiation, and surgery (see "PUBLICATIONS AND TAPES" section below).

When seeking relief for pain, try to be as specific as possible in describing it.

• Is the pain dull or sharp?
• Is it steady or throbbing? Use a scale from 1 to 10 to indicate its intensity, increasing the number as the pain increases.
• If the pain is constant, is it more intense at one time of day than another?
• How long does the current pain medication work?
• Do any normal activities increase or decrease the pain? Keep a diary of these details.

If your doctor is unable to offer you a pain relief method that works, ask for a referral to a pain specialist. Good sources for information about cancer pain control are the local hospital's oncology department, a hospice, or cancer center (often a specialty hospital or section of a general or teaching hospital). The American Cancer Society and the National Cancer Institute offer toll-free telephone hotlines and web sites that can direct consumers to pain specialists (see "ORGANIZATIONS" section below).

References

Bates, David W.
1997   "The Costs of Adverse Drug Events in Hospitalized Patients" JAMA 277:4(January 22-29):307-311
Bates, David W. et al.
1999   "Patient Risk Factors for Adverse Drug Events in Hospitalized Patients" Archives of Internal Medicine 159(November):2553-2560
Bates, David W. et al.
1998   "Effect of a Computerized Physician Order Entry and a Team Intervention on Prevention of Serious Medication Errors" JAMA 280:15(October 21):1311-1316
Desbiens, N.A. et al.
1996   "Pain and Satisfaction with Pain Control in Seriously Ill Hospitalized Adults: Findings from the SUPPORT Research Investigations" Critical Care Medicine 24:12(December):1953-1961
Fields, Howard L. and Joseph B. Martin
1994   "Pain: Pathophysiology and Management" pp. 49-55 in Kurt J. Isselbacher et al. (eds.) Harrison's Principles of Internal Medicine New York, NY: McGraw-Hill Inc.
Food and Drug Administration
1996   "The Clinical Impact of Adverse Event Reporting" MedWatch October
1995   "Clinical Therapeutics and the Recognition of Drug-Induced Disease" MedWatch Continuing Education Article
Honaker, Ann
1995   "Impasse in Pain Management: The Case of Parkland Memorial Hospital" The Picker Report 3:1:(Winter):3, 6

Leape, Lucian L. et al.
1995 "Systems Analysis of Adverse Drug Events" <u>JAMA</u> 274:1(July 5):35-43
Levin, M.L., J.I. Berry, and J. Leiter
1998 "Management of Pain in Terminally Ill Patients: Physician Reports of Knowledge, Attitudes, and Behavior" <u>Journal of Pain Symptom Management</u> 15:1(January):27-40
Walker, Janice D.
1995 "Enhancing Physical Comfort in the Hospital" <u>The Picker Report</u> 3:1:(Winter):1-2, 5

ORGANIZATIONS

American Cancer Society (ACS)
1599 Clifton Road, NE
Atlanta, GA 30329
(800) 227-2345   www.cancer.org

This national voluntary health organization funds research and provides education, advocacy, and services to individuals with cancer, their families, and professionals. Local affiliates throughout the country.

American Chronic Pain Association (ACPA)
PO Box 850
Rocklin, CA 95677
(916) 632-0922   FAX (916) 632-3208
e-mail: acpa@pacbell.net   www.theacpa.org

Organizes groups throughout the U.S. to provide support and activities for people who experience chronic pain. Membership, $30.00 first year, $15.00 thereafter; includes quarterly newsletter, "ACPA Chronicle."

American Pain Foundation (APF)
201 North Charles Street, Suite 710
Baltimore, MD 2120
(888) 615-7246   FAX (410) 385-1832
e-mail: info@painfoundation.org   www.painfoundation.org

This organization provides educational materials and advocates on behalf of people who are experiencing pain. It promotes research and advocates to remove barriers to treatment for pain. It distributes patient educational materials (free) and has information about the causes of pain and treatment as well as links to related sites on its web site.

American Pain Society (APS)
4700 West Lake Avenue
Glen View, IL 60025
(847) 375-4715   FAX (877) 734-8758
e-mail: info@ampainsoc.org   www.ampainsoc.org

The Society is a multidisciplinary membership organization that has the goals of advancing research, education, and professional services for people in pain. Membership dues for professionals vary by income level from $100.00 to $235.00. Individual membership, $125.00. Membership includes the quarterly publication "The Journal of Pain" and a newsletter, the "APS Bulletin." Users may search a database of pain treatment facilities on the web site.

American Society of Anesthesiologists (ASA)
520 North Northwest Highway
Park Ridge, IL 60068
(847) 825-5586   FAX (847) 825-1692   www.asahq.org

A professional membership organization for anesthesiologists. Publishes patient education brochures such as "Know Your Anesthesiologist," "Anesthesia for Ambulatory Surgery," "When Your Child Needs Anesthesia," and "The Senior Citizen as a Patient." Single copy, free.

City of Hope Pain/Palliative Care Resource Center
1500 East Duarte Road
Duarte, CA 91010
(626) 359-8111, extension 63829   FAX (626) 301-8941
e-mail: mayday-pain@coh.org   mayday.coh.org

This national clearinghouse provides information on pain management for individuals and professionals. A Resource List that include organizations, videotapes, audiocassettes, and print publications is available free plus $3.00 shipping and handling. Also available on the web site.

Commission on Accreditation of Rehabilitation Facilities (CARF)
4891 East Grant Road
Tucson, AZ 85712
(520) 325-1044 (V/TT)   FAX (520) 318-1129
e-mail: webmaster@carf.org   www.carf.org

Will provide a free list of inpatient and outpatient facilities that have accredited acute, chronic, and cancer pain management programs in a single state.

Food and Drug Administration (FDA)
5600 Fishers Lane
Rockville, MD 20857
(888) 463-6332   (301) 827-4420   FAX (301) 443-9767
e-mail: execsec@oc.fda.gov   www.fda.gov

This federal agency is responsible for approving new drugs before they enter the market. Publishes "FDA Consumer," a newsletter that reports on food safety, medical devices, drugs, blood products, cosmetics, vaccines, nutrition, radiation protection, and veterinary medicine; $13.50 (six issues); free on FDA's web site, which includes back issues and index. Free sample available upon request.

Institute for Safe Medication Practices (ISMP)
1800 Byberry Road, Suite 819
Huntington Valley, PA 19006
(215) 947-7797   FAX (215) 914-1492
e-mail: ismpinfo@ismp.org   www.ismp.org

Provides assistance to callers regarding medication errors and medication error prevention methods. Maintain reference articles covering this subject. Administers the Medication Errors Reporting Program, which enables health care professionals to report medication errors or potential errors. Web site includes information about medical alerts and links to other sites.

Joint Commission on Accreditation of Healthcare Organizations (JCAHO)
1 Renaissance Boulevard
Oakbrook Terrace, IL 60181
(630) 792-5000   FAX (630) 792-5005   www.jcaho.org

This organization provides accreditation to health care organizations including hospitals, home care, long term care, and ambulatory care facilities. The health care facilities must pay for the accreditation survey. Criteria used for accreditation evaluations are described on the web site and in JCAHO publications. Beginning in 2001, JCAHO will be issuing scores for compliance with its pain management standards. JCAHO has a consumer information section on its web site, where it is possible to find the accreditation status of specific facilities. Consumers may file complaints about facilities by phoning (800) 994-6610 or e-mailing to complaint@jcaho.org. Consumer publications such as "Helping You Choose The Hospital for You" and "Helping You Choose A Quality Health Plan" are available. Single copy, free. Also available on the web site.

The Mayday Fund
c/o UBS-AG
10 East 50th Street
New York, NY 10022
(212) 838-2904   www.painandhealth.org/mayday/mayday-home.html

The goal of the Mayday Fund is to close the gap between the knowledge about pain control and current medical practice regarding pain control. Projects that aim to improve public policy regarding pain control, those using multidisciplinary personnel, and those related to children's pain will be considered for funding. Contact the Fund for an application.

MedWatch
Food and Drug Administration (FDA)
5600 Fishers Lane
Rockville, MD 20852
(800) 332-1088   FAX (800) 332-0178   (301) 443-0117
www.fda.gov/medwatch

The Medical Products Reporting Program reports safety warnings and recalls for products regulated by the FDA, such as drugs, medical devices, devices that emit radiation, special nutritional products, and biologics (blood, etc.). Users may access the information online. Health professionals and consumers are encouraged to report problems with the use of any of these products to Medwatch. MedWatch distributes free e-mail notices regarding problems in drugs and medical products. Sign up on the web site.

National Cancer Institute (NCI)
Physician Data Query (PDQ)
CancerNet
CANCERLIT
LiveHelp
31 Center Drive MSC 2580
Building 31, Room 10A03
Bethesda, MD 20892
(800) 422-6237   (800) 332-8615 (TT)   FAX (301) 402-5874
CancerFax (800) 624-2511   e-mail: cancermail@cips.nci.nih.gov
cancer.gov

The National Cancer Institute supports basic and clinical research investigations into the causes, prevention, and cure for cancer. The PDQ database provides up-to-date information on cancer prevention, screening, clinical trials, treatments, and care. PDQ is available on the Internet through CancerNet, which also contains fact sheets and publications, CancerNet news, and CANCERLIT abstracts and citations. CancerFax provides access by fax machine to information statements from the PDQ Database, CANCERLIT citations and abstracts, and fact sheets on cancer topics. LiveHelp is a pilot program that provides live, online assistance from an NCI Information Specialist; available Monday-Friday, 12-4 pm, Eastern Time. Most information is also available in Spanish. Calling the "800" phone number listed above connects with the regional center closest to you, which can provide information about the resources described above as well as local resources.

National Chronic Pain Outreach Association (NCPOA)
PO Box 274
Millboro, VA 24460
(540) 862-9437   FAX (540) 862-9485
e-mail: ncpoa@cfw.com

A national clearinghouse for information about chronic pain. Refers individuals to support groups on chronic pain throughout the U.S. Produces publications and audiocassettes on a variety of topics related to chronic pain. Membership, individuals, $25.00; professionals, $50.00; includes quarterly newsletter, "Lifeline."

National Institutes of Health Consensus Program
PO Box 2577
Kensington, MD 20891
(888) 644-2667   FAX (301) 816-2494
e-mail: consensus_statements@nih.gov
consensus.nih.gov

Sponsors conferences that produce consensus statements on the effectiveness, risks, and clinical applications of biomedical technology. Consensus statements on subjects such as breast cancer screening, kidney dialysis, impotence, epilepsy, pain management, and osteoporosis are available on the web site.

National Organization for Rare Disorders (NORD)
100 Rt. 37, PO Box 8923
New Fairfield, CT 06812-8923
(800) 999-6673   (203) 746-6518   (203) 746-6927 (TT)
FAX (203) 746-6481   e-mail: orphan@rarediseases.org
www.rarediseases.org

Federation of voluntary health organizations that serves individuals with rare or "orphan" diseases. Conducts the Medication Assistance Program. Membership, $30.00. Reprints of articles on rare diseases available from the NORD Rare Disease Database for $7.50 per copy; abstracts available free on web site. Publishes newsletter, "Orphan Disease Update," three times a year; free.

Needy Meds
www.needymeds.com

This web site lists pharmaceutical manufacturers who offer programs to assist individuals who cannot afford drugs prescribed for them. Includes special requirements, procedures, and forms.

Pharmaceutica Information Network
pharminfo.com

This web site enables the user to search specific drugs to learn about their effects, interactions with other drugs, etc. Provides links to other related web sites.

Rxlist
www.rxlist.com

This web site enables the user to search specific drugs to learn about their effects, interactions with other drugs, etc. Provides links to other related web sites.

PUBLICATIONS AND TAPES

<u>Advice for the Patient: Drug Information in Lay Language</u>
Micromedex
6200 South Syracuse Way, Suite 300
Greenwood Village, CO 80111
(800) 877-6209   FAX (201) 722-2680
www.info@mdx.com

This book provides information on prescription drugs and describes precautions and side effects. Includes a glossary and list of poison control centers. $80.00 plus $10.00 shipping and handling

<u>Cancer Pain Treatment Guidelines for Patients</u>
National Comprehensive Cancer Network (NCCN)
50 Huntingdon Pike, Suite 200
Rockledge, PA 19046
(888) 909-6226   (215) 728-4788   FAX (215) 728-3877
e-mail: patientinformation@nccn.org
www.nccn.org/patient/guidelines

These guidelines, developed by the NCCN and the American Cancer Society, are based on NCCN Oncology Practice Guidelines. Available in English and Spanish. Also available on the NCCN web site and the American Cancer Society web site: www.cancer.org

<u>Complete Drug Reference 2001</u>
Consumer Reports Books
PO Box 10637
Des Moines, IA 50336-0637
(800) 500-9760   FAX (515) 237-4765

Indexed by both generic and brand names, this book provides consumers with information on prescription and nonprescription medicines. $44.95 plus $3.50 shipping and handling

<u>Consumers Guide to Cancer Drugs</u>
American Cancer Society (ACS)
NCICFUL
PO Box 102454
Atlanta, GA 30368
(800) 227-2345   www.cancer.org

This book provides information on drugs used to treat cancer and those used to manage symptoms. Lists side effects and describes how the drugs are administered. Includes glossary of treatment terms. $16.95

Controlling Cancer Pain: A Video for Patients and Families
Cancer Information Center, National Cancer Institute (NCI)
31 Center Drive MSC 2580
Building 31, Room 10A03
Bethesda, MD 20892
(800) 422-6237   (800) 332-8615 (TT)   FAX (301) 402-5874
CancerFax (800) 624-2511   e-mail: cancermail@cips.nci.nih.gov
cancer.gov

In this videotape, three individuals describe the pain management techniques they use. Includes oral and intravenous medications and patient controlled analgesia (PCA). Closed captioned. 12 minutes. Free

Directory of Prescription Drug Patient Assistance Programs
Pharmaceutical Research and Manufacturers Association (PHRMA)
1100 15th Street, NW
Washington, DC 20005
(800) 762-4636   (202) 835-3400   www.phrma.org

A list of members that offer certain drugs at low or no cost to uninsured or underinsured patients. Most programs require that a physician make the request. Free

FDA's Tips for Taking Medicines: How to Get the Most Benefits with the Fewest Risks
by Dixie Farley
Food and Drug Administration (FDA)
5600 Fishers Lane, HFI-40
Rockville, MD 20857
(888) 463-6332   (301) 827-4420   FAX (301) 443-9767
www.fda.gov

This article suggests questions to ask when new medications are prescribed and describes medication counseling available to consumers. Free. Also available on the web site.

Management of Cancer Pain
Clinical Practice Guideline, Number 9
Agency for Healthcare Research and Quality Publications Clearinghouse
PO Box 8547
Silver Spring, MD 20907-8547
(800) 358-9295   (888) 586-6340 (TT)   e-mail: info@ahrq.gov
www.ahrq.gov

This guideline for clinicians provides recommendations about the assessment and management of pain and describes methods for pharmacologic and nonpharmacologic management.

Includes section on managing pain in special populations such as infants, children, adolescents, elders, and patients with AIDS. Free. Also available on the web site.

Managing Cancer Pain
Agency for Healthcare Research and Quality Publications Clearinghouse
PO Box 8547
Silver Spring, MD 20907-8547
(800) 358-9295   (888) 586-6340 (TT)   e-mail: info@ahrq.gov
www.ahrq.gov

This booklet describes various treatments available for cancer pain, including drugs, relaxation exercises, and other nonmedical treatments. Includes pain control record form. Free. Also available on the web site.

Pain Control After Surgery: A Patient's Guide
Agency for Healthcare Research and Quality Publications Clearinghouse
PO Box 8547
Silver Spring, MD 20907-8547
(800) 358-9295   (888) 586-6340 (TT)   e-mail: info@ahrq.gov
www.ahrq.gov

This booklet suggests questions to ask about pain control before surgery and discusses a pain control plan. Describes pain relief medications and nondrug pain relief methods. Free. Also available on the web site.

Pain Control: A Guide for People with Cancer and Their Families
American Cancer Society (ACS)
1599 Clifton Road, NE
Atlanta, GA 30329
(800) 227-2345   www.cancer.org

This booklet describes prescription and nonprescription pain relievers, nondrug treatments, and other techniques for pain control. Includes daily pain diary. Free

Pain in the Elderly
by Betty R. Ferrell and Bruce A. Ferrell (eds.)
IASP Press
909 NE 43rd Street, Suite 306
Seattle, WA 98105
(206) 547-6409   FAX (206) 547-1703
e-mail: iaspbooks@juno.com   www.painbooks.org

This book discusses acute and chronic pain in elders and the complications of multiple medical problems and treatment related side effects. $25.00

Pain Management
Films for the Humanities and Sciences
PO Box 2053
Princeton, NJ 08543
(800) 257-5126   FAX (609) 275-3767
e-mail: custserv@films.com   www.films.com

This videotape portrays patients who are recovering from surgery, living with cancer pain, or coping with chronic pain. Physicians discuss various methods of pain control. 28 minutes. Purchase, $129.00; rental, $75.00; plus 6% shipping and handling.

PDR Family Guide to Prescription Drugs
Random House
400 Hahn Road
Westminster, MD 21157
(800) 733-3000   (410) 848-1900   FAX (410) 386-7013
www.randomhouse.com

This book provides drug profiles arranged by brand name and cross referenced to generic versions. Also includes overviews of major health problems and treatments. $23.00 plus $5.50 shipping and handling

The People's Pharmacy
by Joe Graedon and Teresa Gradeon
St. Martin's Press
c/o VHPS
16365 James Madison Highway
Gordonsville, VA 22940
(800) 321-9299   www.stmartins.com

This book provides general information on prescription medicines, over-the-counter drugs, and home remedies as well as instructions, side effects, interactions and other precautions for many commonly prescribed medications. $16.95

Physicians' Desk Reference (PDR) $86.95
Physicians' Desk Reference for Nonprescription Drugs and Dietary Supplements $58.95
Medical Economics Company
PO Box 10689
Des Moines, IA 50336-0689
(800) 678-5689   FAX (515) 284-6714

This series of drug reference books provides detailed information about prescription and over-the-counter drugs. Uses technical format approved by the Food and Drug Administration. Includes full text of each product's government approved labeling.

Prescription Medicines and You: A Consumer Guide
Agency for Healthcare Research and Quality Publications Clearinghouse
PO Box 8547
Silver Spring, MD 20907-8547
(800) 358-9295   (888) 586-6340 (TT)   e-mail: info@ahrq.gov
www.ahrq.gov

This booklet enables consumers to become involved in their treatment plans and ask appropriate questions when talking with physicians, nurses, and pharmacists about their prescription medication. Available in English, Spanish, and Asian languages. Free. Also available at the web site by clicking on "Consumer Health."

20 Tips to Help Prevent Medical Errors
Agency for Healthcare Research and Quality Publications Clearinghouse
PO Box 8547
Silver Spring, MD 20907-8547
(800) 358-9295   (888) 586-6340 (TT)   e-mail: info@ahrq.gov
www.ahrq.gov

This brochure provides tips for discussing medications with doctors, pharmacists, and hospital personnel in order to prevent medical errors. Free

Understanding Cancer Pain
Cancer Information Center, National Cancer Institute (NCI)
31 Center Drive MSC 2580
Building 31, Room 10A03
Bethesda, MD 20892
(800) 422-6237   (800) 332-8615 (TT)   FAX (301) 402-5874
CancerFax (800) 624-2511   e-mail: cancermail@cips.nci.nih.gov
cancer.gov

This booklet describes methods used to control cancer pain and provides a pain rating scale and pain diary. Large print. Available in English and Spanish. Also available on the web site.

Worst Pills, Best Pills
Public Citizen Health Research Group
1600 20th Street, NW
Washington, DC 20009
(202) 588-1000   www.citizen.org

This book provides information on 119 drugs that are dangerous and 245 safer alternatives. $16.00

<u>Worst Pills, Best Pills News</u>
Public Citizen Health Research Group
1600 20th Street, NW
Washington, DC 20009
(202) 588-1000   www.citizen.org

A monthly newsletter that provides the latest information about prescription and over-the-counter drugs, suggestions for avoiding drugs on the market without proper warning labels, and warnings about potentially dangerous drug interactions. $20.00

Chapter 7

PROTECTING THE HEALTH OF CHILDREN WHO ARE ILL

When a child becomes seriously ill, parents may become very emotional. It is at this very time, however, when they need to remain rational so that they may ensure that the child receives optimal health care. Parents make the medical care decisions for their children except in emergencies or if a court has ordered treatment to save the child's life. In addition to the wide range of resources available to anyone making a medical decision, there are special resources and support groups to help parents cope with a child's illness. In cases where child abuse is suspected, parents may be excluded from an examination room, but an adult witness should be present. "Informed consent" for minors means that the parent or guardian must give permission for medical treatment or surgical procedures.

The *Health Insurance Portability and Accountability Act (HIPAA) of 1996* (P.L. 104-191), described in Chapter 5, also required the Department of Health and Human Services to develop regulations to protect the privacy of individuals' medical records. The regulations went into effect on April 14, 2001. Under HIPAA's privacy rules, parents serve as the personal representatives of their minor children and have the right to obtain their health information. Exceptions occur when state or other law does not require parental consent for a minor to receive a particular health care service or when a court authorizes someone else to make the minor's health decisions.

SELECTING A PEDIATRICIAN

Maintaining an ongoing relationship with a physician you trust and have confidence in is extremely valuable, whether a child was born with a serious illness or develops one later in childhood. This relationship provides a potential link with referrals to specialists and health care facilities. Use the same criteria in choosing a pediatrician for your child as you would in choosing your own primary care physician. Consider the following in selecting a pediatrician:

> • Did we get an appointment within a reasonable amount of time?
> • Did we have to wait too long in the pediatrician's office?
> • Did the pediatrician conduct the examination, or did a nurse practitioner or physician assistant conduct the examination?
> • Did the pediatrician treat us with respect? What tone of voice did he or she use with our child? Does our child like the physician?
> • Did the pediatrician encourage us to ask questions? Did he or she answer them to our satisfaction? Or did the pediatrician feel threatened by our questions and say that we did not need the information we requested? Did he or she seem distracted and not able to concentrate on our concerns?
> • Did the exam seem thorough?

• Did the pediatrician explain what he or she was going to do next during the exam both to us and to our child? Did he or she calm our child's fears during the exam?

• Was someone available to watch our child after the examination so that we could talk alone with the pediatrician?

• Did the pediatrician describe the diagnosis in clear terms and make certain that we understood it?

• Did the pediatrician pay adequate attention to our emotional responses to the diagnosis of a serious condition? Did he or she recognize our grief in learning that our child has a life long condition/disability?

• Did the pediatrician present alternative treatment options and then seek out our opinion?

• Did the pediatrician provide thorough instructions for using a prescription drug, including information about interactions with other drugs or food and information about side effects?

• Does the pediatrician's approach to medical treatment seem compatible with ours, i.e., does he or she take a wait-and-see approach or a more aggressive approach?

• Did the pediatrician phone us promptly with the results of lab tests? Did he or she send us copies of our child's test results when we requested them? Did he or she provide a written interpretation of the results with suggestions for treatment?

• How did the pediatrician respond to our request to seek a second opinion? If the response was positive, were any recommendations made? Were the recommended pediatricians part of the same practice?

• Who covers for the pediatrician when he or she is unavailable? (Parents should meet the pediatricians who cover.)

• Does the pediatrician have "calling hours" so that we can ask questions or discuss our concerns?

• How comfortable is the pediatrician in explaining our child's condition to him or her?

• Does the pediatrician acknowledge that our child is part of a family and that other family members' needs must also be addressed?

• Is the pediatrician's office staff cooperative, returning phone calls and filling out forms required by education or service organizations?

A classic study by Korsch and her colleagues (1968) found that pediatricians often ignore mothers' questions or give vague answers. Quite understandably, mothers who did not have their questions answered satisfactorily were not likely to follow through on the medical advice given by the pediatricians. Should you find yourself in this situation, repeat your questions to the pediatrician. If the pediatrician still ignores you or gives a vague, unsatisfactory answer, make clear that you feel communications could be improved, and ask for literature on the topic. If the pediatrician seems unwilling to respond to your request, it is time to seek out a new pediatrician.

MAINTAINING MEDICAL RECORDS
(Also see Chapter 1, "Keeping A Journal of Your Medical History" section)

Parents should keep their own set of records of their children's medical histories, including symptoms, diagnostic test results, diagnoses, and treatments. Note any allergies or side effects from drugs. Request copies of all test results.

Keeping this information up-to-date and organized will prove helpful when seeing new physicians or filling out insurance or hospital admission forms. When a child is seriously ill, it is helpful to keep a daily journal or calendar, recording medical appointments, lab tests and results, and medications. This information might also be kept on tape or in computer files. These details are especially important when dealing with hospital billing departments and insurance companies.

IF YOUR CHILD HAS A DISABILITY OR CHRONIC CONDITION

Managing the care of a child with a disability or chronic condition is a major responsibility for parents. For some parents, it may become overwhelming. But if parents can channel their anxiety into productive actions by learning as much as possible about their child's condition, they will contribute to providing optimal medical care.

In addition to asking the usual questions all parents should ask when selecting a new pediatrician, parents of a child with a disability or chronic condition must ask questions related to the child's conditions and the pediatrician's experience in treating the conditions.

> • How many other children with special needs do you see in the practice?
> • How many children with the same condition as your child has the pediatrician treated?
> • Does the pediatrician feel comfortable dealing with the condition?
> • Does the hospital where the pediatrician practices offer special services to children with disabilities and their families?
> • Does the pediatrician have a cooperative relationship with other physicians who may be needed to treat a child with this condition?

Noting that several studies have documented that pediatricians have been lacking in their role as case managers for children who are chronically ill, McInerny (1984) makes numerous recommendations to improve the situation. Included are the need to understand the family's strengths and weaknesses in order to help them build upon their strengths; to discuss with the parents how to inform the child about his or her condition; and to make referrals to service providers such as nurse practitioners and social workers as well as parent support groups.

The professional's responsibility to the family goes far beyond initial discussions of a disability or chronic condition. One study found that parents expressed dissatisfaction with the behavior of physicians and other health care professionals who had not provided the assistance and information needed for making informed decisions about their children's care (Davis: 1991). Parents expressed the need to be treated with respect, to be spoken to in an unpatronizing manner, to have their expertise as parents acknowledged, and to have their family as a whole considered.

Because parents experience such intense emotional reactions to a child's illness or disability, counseling may help in coping with emotions and contribute to helping the child. Such counseling may be available from medical professionals, social workers or psychologists, rehabilitation counselors, and other parents in similar situations. Talking with other parents either in private or at a parent support group helps parents to learn that their emotional responses are normal. Parent groups also serve as a mechanism to channel energy into productive ways of helping the child. Support groups, which in many cases are focused on a specific disability or disease, help parents learn about the services available for the child and how to interact effectively with a variety of professionals. In addition to providing information and referrals, parent groups may also have a system of providing respite care.

Although numerous professionals may be involved in helping children with disabilities and chronic conditions, ultimately it is the parents' responsibility to ensure that their child receives optimal medical care, rehabilitation, and education. Gliedman and Roth make several suggestions to help parents achieve this goal, including:

- Monitor your child's progress closely and keep copies of your child's records.
- Keep records of visits with professionals, including dates, who was present, and what was said.
- If you do not understand any terms that are used, ask for a translation into lay language.
- Learn as much as you can about your child's condition.
- Listen to your child when he or she expresses individual needs.
(1980: 184-185)

At a symposium, parents whose children had sustained traumatic injuries, physicians, and other health care professionals recommended training for physicians to help them deliver crucial information accurately, sensitively, and understandably (Lash: 1995). Recognizing the difficulties in maintaining clear channels of communication as children are moved from the emergency room to intensive care or perhaps transferred to a regional trauma center, they suggested supplementing family meetings with concrete tools such as a family notebook, check lists, and written practical information.

In their study of families whose children were diagnosed with Down syndrome, congenital heart disease, or both conditions, Garwick and colleagues found that their reactions to these diagnoses were influenced by the setting in which the news was given, pre-existing family factors, characteristics of the condition, and the strategy used to provide information.

Families remember learning about their child's condition as though it were yesterday. Often they can tell you what they were wearing, the exact words the physicians used. They remember the room. But most of all, they remember how they felt. They remember their emotions. (Garwick et al.: 1995)

LAWS THAT AFFECT CHILDREN'S HEALTH CARE

In 1997, Congress passed the *Children's Health Insurance Program* (P.L. 105-33), part of the Balanced Budget Act of 1997), CHIP, to make available funds for states to provide insurance for uninsured children of low income, working parents. States have the option of expanding their Medicaid plan or developing a new children's health insurance plan. States are required to submit a plan for approval to the Secretary of Health and Human Services; the law sets standards for what the coverage must include. Eligibility requirements for the program are an income level 200 percent of the poverty level or 50 percentage points above the Medicaid eligibility limit; and children must not be eligible for Medicaid or other health insurance coverage. States must continue Medicaid eligibility for children who would have lost SSI benefits because of the change in the definition of childhood disability under the Personal Responsibility and Work Opportunity Act of 1996.

The *Family Opportunity Act of 2001* would allow states to offer a Medicaid buy-in for children with disabilities up to age 18 who would be eligible for SSI disability benefits but for their family income. This plan would cover children whose families earn up to 300% of the federal poverty level ($52,950 for a family of four). As this book went to press, the 106th Congress had not completed action on the bill before adjournment.

PREPARING YOUR CHILD FOR MEDICAL PROCEDURES OR SURGERY

It is important for parents to understand their child's developmental stage when they are preparing their child for a medical examination, test, or surgery. Children under the age of three are very anxious when separated from their parents and should be reassured that Mommy/Daddy will return. Children ages four to seven are more likely to fear mutilation or loss of a body part. If an operation is scheduled, children need to be told what will happen to them. Booklets written especially for youngsters can help demystify the upcoming experience. Medical personnel may use anatomically correct teaching dolls to demonstrate medical procedures such as blood drawing, giving intravenous medication, catheterization, or setting a fracture. Children ages eight to 12 who are building their self-confidence may benefit from a tour of the outpatient surgery center, so that they may ask questions for themselves and feel that they have some control over the situation. There are a number of age-appropriate books to read together in preparation for surgery or a hospital stay (see "PUBLICATIONS AND TAPES" section below). Familiar objects such as a stuffed animal, a favorite blanket, or family pictures may help a child feel more comfortable in unfamiliar surroundings. Research has shown that children who are prepared for surgery are less fearful, more cooperative, and recover better (Brazelton: 1996).

Hospital admission procedures are the same for a child as for an adult, although parents should act as the child's advocate. Obtain the following information when your child is scheduled to enter a hospital:

- The purpose of each test required by the hospital prior to admission.
- The type of anesthesia that is planned, its side effects, and dosage. Is the dosage determined by the child's body weight? Has it been evaluated for use in children? How long after the surgery will it have lingering effects?
- Other medications that will be used and what their side effects are
- A description of the surgery.
- The hospital's policy about permitting parents to accompany their child

When surgery is completed, the child will be moved to the recovery room, then to a post-surgical area to be reunited with his or her parents. Before leaving this area, parents should be certain that they have received information about pain medication, diet, and restriction on activities.

Several unique characteristics affect pain control in children, including their parents' or caregivers' perception of the need for pain medication and a child's fear of injections. A child's inability to describe or quantify pain may require special assessment techniques. Children as young as eight may use a small computerized pump to administer pain medication (American Society of Anesthesiologists: 1994).

Less than one-fifth of the drugs available in the marketplace have been evaluated for use in children (National Organization for Rare Disorders: 1998). This means that pediatricians receive no information about side effects or dosage recommendations for the antibiotics, stimulants, antidepressants, and pain control medications they prescribe for their patients. In 1998, the Food and Drug Administration proposed a rule that would require drug companies to include children in clinical trials of new drugs. Drugs that are currently used in treating children must also be studied.

Adverse drug events are not uncommon in pediatric inpatient settings. In a recent study, Kaushal and colleagues (2001) examined the pediatric medication orders, administration records, and patient charts over a six week period at two major metropolitan hospitals. They suggested that an error rate of nearly six percent could have been prevented by a computerized physician order system and the presence of onsite pediatric pharmacists. Parents can help protect their children by asking, before any injection or pill is administered, "What is this drug? What is it for?" Hospital personnel should always check your child's identification bracelet to ascertain that he or she is the intended recipient. The wristband should list your child's drug allergies. Although you may tire of endless questions about drug allergies asked by all personnel who enter your child's hospital room, answer them carefully and thoroughly. Take note of any changes in your child's condition and report them to the medical staff.

References

American Society of Anesthesiologists
1994 <u>When Your Child Needs Anesthesia</u> Park Ridge, IL: American Society of Anesthesiologists

Brazelton, T. Berry
1996 <u>Going to the Doctor</u> Reading, MA: Addison-Wesley-Longman Publishing Company

Davis, Hilton
1991 "Counselling Families of Children with Disabilities" pp. 223-37 in Hilton Davis and Lesley Fallowfield (eds.) <u>Counselling and Communication in Health Care</u> London: John Wiley & Sons

Garwick, Ann W. et al.
1995 "Breaking the News: How Families First Learn About Their Child's Chronic Condition" <u>Archives of Pediatrics & Adolescent Medicine</u> 149:9(September):991-997

Gliedman, John and William Roth
1980 <u>The Unexpected Minority: Handicapped Children in America</u> New York, NY: Harcourt Brace Jovanovich

Kaushal, Rainu et al.
2001 "Medication Errors and Adverse Drug Events in Pediatric Inpatients" <u>JAMA</u> 285:16(April 25):2114-2120

Korsch, Barbara et al.
1968 "Gaps in Doctor Patient Interactions and Patient Satisfaction" <u>Pediatrics</u> 43:855-870

Lash, Marilyn
1995 "How Can Parents and Professionals Communicate Effectively?" <u>REHAB Update</u> Fall 1995/Winter 1995 pp. 6-7

McInerny, Thomas
1984 "The Role of the General Pediatrician in Coordinating the Care of Children with Chronic Illness" <u>Pediatric Clinics of North America</u> 31(February)1:199-209

National Organization for Rare Disorders
1998 <u>Orphan Disease Update</u> 15:3:4

ORGANIZATIONS

American Academy of Pediatrics (AAP)
141 Northwest Point Boulevard
Elk Grove Village, IL 60007
(888) 443-9016   FAX (847) 434-8000
e-mail: kidsdocs@aap.org   www.aap.org

A professional membership society for pediatricians, this organization publishes the monthly journal "Pediatrics," which is available in print ($130.00) or on their web site. It is possible to view the table of contents, abstracts, e-mail alerts, and full text articles in "Pediatrics" electronic pages at no cost. The AAP also publishes a variety of guides for parents related to different stages of a child's life.

Children's Oncology Group (COG)
440 East Huntington Drive, Suite 300
Arcadia, CA 91006
(626) 447-0064   FAX (626) 445-4334   www.nccf.org/cog

This collaborative national pediatric research group conducts clinical trials of new therapies for childhood cancer.

Family Voices
3411 Candelaria NE, Suite M
Albuquerque, NM 87107
(888) 835-5669   (505) 872-4774   FAX (505) 872-4780
e-mail: kidshealth@familyvoices.org
www.familyvoices.org

This national grassroots network of families has developed a wide range of projects to improve health care for children with disabilities. These projects include the development of health education materials that promote family involvement in state children's health insurance programs, connecting children with disabilities and chronic conditions with one another, and advocacy in public policy areas such as special education, managed care, employment, and health care. Membership is free. Bimonthly newsletter, "Family Voices," $25.00. Available in English and Spanish. "Friday's Child," is a weekly newsletter sent by e-mail and fax. It provides information about legislation, conferences, and other announcements.

KidsHealth
www.kidshealth.org

This web site, sponsored by the Nemours Foundation, provides health information for children, adolescents, and parents. Includes links for topics such as going to the hospital, having surgery and getting tests, dealing with feelings, and a glossary of medical terms.

National Information Center for Children and Youth with Disabilities (NICHCY)
PO Box 1492
Washington, DC 20013-1492
(800) 695-0285 (V/TT)   In the Washington, DC area, (202) 884-8200 (V/TT)
FAX (202) 884-8441   e-mail: nichcy@aed.org
www.nichcy.org

Provides information and referral, technical assistance, and publications to parents, educators, caregivers, and advocates. Publications are available on the web site.

Pediatric Database
www.icondata.com/health/pedbase/index.htm

Designed by a pediatrician, this database provides information on more than 550 pediatric disorders. The entire database may be downloaded.

Shriner's Hospitals for Children
2900 Rocky Point Drive
Tampa, FL 33607
(800) 237-5055   (813) 281-0300   www.shrinershq.org

Provides free medical care for children with orthopedic problems, spinal cord injuries, and burns. Twenty-two hospitals are located in the U.S., Canada, and Mexico.

Starbright Foundation
11835 West Olympic Boulevard, Suite 500
Los Angeles, CA 90064
(800) 315-2580   (310) 479-1212   FAX (310) 479-1235
www.starbright.org

This organization uses technology to develop projects for seriously ill children, including a diabetes game on CD-ROM and videotapes that address medical and emotional needs (see "PUBLICATIONS AND TAPES" section below). It also sponsors "Starbright World," a private computer network for children and adolescents who are chronically or seriously ill, so that they may interact with peers in the U.S. and Canada. Free

St. Jude Children's Research Hospital
501 St. Jude Place
Memphis, TN 38105-1942
(800) 877-5833   (901) 578-2000   www.stjude.org

Provides free care for children with catastrophic illnesses such as genetic diseases, cancer, and immunodeficient conditions.

Advice to Doctors and Other Big People from Kids
Celestial Arts Publishing Company
PO Box 7123
Berkeley, CA 94707
(800) 841-2665   (510) 554-1600   FAX (510) 559-1629
www.tenspeed.com

In this book, children with life-threatening illnesses discuss medical exams, hospitalization, talking with medical professionals, going through treatment, and advice to other children and their families. $7.95 plus $4.50 shipping and handling

American Medical Association Complete Guide to Your Children's Health
Random House
400 Hahn Road
Westminster, MD 21157
(800) 733-3000   (410) 848-1900   FAX (410) 386-7013
www.randomhouse.com

This book covers the health needs of children from infancy through adolescence. Includes sections on choosing a pediatrician; routine tests and screenings; first aid and emergency care; symptom charts; and helping children with special health needs. $39.95 plus $5.50 shipping and handling

Blueberry Eyes
by Monica Driscoll Beatty
Health Press
PO Drawer 1388
Santa Fe, NM 87504
(505) 474-0303   FAX (505) 424-0444   www.healthpress.com

This children's book describes the experiences of a seven year old who has eye surgery. $8.95 plus $4.00 shipping and handling

Bright Futures Family Pocket Guide: Raising Healthy Infants, Children and Adolescents
Family Voices at the Federation for Children with Special Needs
1135 Tremont Street, Suite 420
Boston, MA 02120
(617) 236-7210 V/TT   FAX (617) 572-2094   www.fcsn.org

This guide offers suggestions for choosing and working with health care providers and describes what to expect at each health care visit. $2.40

Child Health Guide: Put Prevention into Practice
Agency for Healthcare Research and Quality Publications Clearinghouse
PO Box 8547
Silver Spring, MD 20907
(800) 358-9295   (888) 586-6340 (TT)   e-mail: info@ahrq.gov
www.ahrq.gov

This pocket-sized guide enables parents or other family members to record their child's important medical care details such as medication records, immunizations, and preventative tests. Free. Also available on the web site.

Children with Disabilities: A Medical Primer
Mark L. Batshaw and Yvonne M. Perret
Brookes Publishing Company
PO Box 10624
Baltimore, MD 21285-9945
(800) 638-3775   FAX (410) 337-8539
e-mail: custserv@pbrookes.com   www.brookespublishing.com

Written by a physician and a social worker, this book describes major types of disability in children, such as hearing impairments, vision impairments, seizure disorders, traumatic brain injury, and AIDS, and provides a glossary and resource list. $59.95 plus 10% shipping and handling

Coping with a Hospital Stay
by Sharon Carter and Judy Monnig
Rosen Publishing Group, Inc.
29 East 21st Street
New York, NY 10010
(800) 237-9932   FAX (888) 436-4643
e-mail: info@rosenpub.com   www.rosenpub.com

Starting with a visit to the emergency room, the authors describe a stay in the hospital. For children ages 7 to 12. $25.25; $18.95 if purchased through the web site.

Clifford Visits the Hospital, $3.25
Curious George Goes to the Hospital, $3.50
Mr. Rogers: Going to the Doctor, $3.95
Scholastic
PO Box 7502
Jefferson City, MO 65102
(800) 724-6527   e-mail: custserv@scholastic.com
www.scholastic.com

These books follow popular children's book characters in medical settings. Shipping and handling, 9% (minimum of $2.25).

Doctors, Disabilities, and the Family: A Parent's Guide
by Suzanne Ripley
National Information Center for Children and Youth with Disabilities (NICHCY)
PO Box 1492
Washington, DC 20013-1492
(800) 695-0285 (V/TT)   In the Washington, DC area, (202) 884-8200 (V/TT)
FAX (202) 844-8441   e-mail: nichcy@aed.org   www.nichcy.org

This guide offers suggestions for choosing a doctor, such as interviewing, discussing a child's special needs, preparing for the first visit, and parents' responsibilities. Includes a list of sample questions on subjects such as medications, tests, referrals, surgery, and hospitalization. $2.00 NICHCY publications are also available on the web site.

Everything You Need to Know About Staying in the Hospital
by Patricia J. Murphy
Rosen Publishing Group, Inc.
29 East 21st Street
New York, NY 10010
(800) 237-9932   FAX (888) 436-4643
e-mail: info@rosenpub.com   www.rosenpub.com

Written for teenagers, this book describes preparations for entering the hospital, provides information about hospital personnel and procedures, and discusses surgery and discharge from the hospital. Includes glossary and resource list. $23.95

Going to the Doctor
by T. Berry Brazelton
Addison-Wesley-Longman Publishing Company

Written for children, this book provides a step-by-step guide to visiting the pediatrician. Describes the procedures used to examine various parts of the body. Includes advice for parents on preparing a child for a doctor's visit. Out of print

Health Care Visit Checklist for Children with Special Health Care Needs
Family Voices
3411 Candelaria NE, Suite M
Albuquerque, NM 87107
(888) 835-5669   (505) 872-4774   FAX (505) 872-4780
e-mail: kidshealth@familyvoices.org
www.familyvoices.org

This fact sheet makes recommendations for preparing for health care visits and suggests questions to ask after the visit. Free. Also available on the web site.

Hospital Stays for Injured Children: Practical Tips for Families
National Pediatric Trauma Registry
New England Medical Center Hospitals, Tufts University School of Medicine
750 Washington Street, Box #75H
Boston, MA 02111
(617) 636-5031 (V/TT)   FAX (617) 636-5513   www.nptr.org

This brochure offers suggestions for the child being hospitalized, the parents, and siblings. Includes checklist of questions to ask before discharge and an information organizer for recordkeeping. Available in English and Spanish. Single copy, free.

Introduction to Managed Care for Children with Special Health Care Needs
Family Voices
3411 Candelaria NE, Suite M
Albuquerque, NM 87107
(888) 835-5669   (505) 872-4774   FAX (505) 872-4780
e-mail: kidshealth@familyvoices.org
www.familyvoices.org

This brochure provides basic information about managed care. Free

Let's Talk About Going to the Doctor
Let's Talk About Going to the Hospital
by Marianne Johnston
PowerKids Press
Rosen Publishing Group, Inc.
29 East 21st Street
New York, NY 10010
(800) 237-9932   FAX (888) 436-4643
e-mail: info@rosenpub.com   www.rosenpub.com

The simple text in these books helps prepare children, ages 2 to 5, for medical care. $17.25; $12.95 if purchased through the web site.

Loving Hands: Homecare for Children
Aquarius Health Care Videos
5 Powderhouse Lane
PO Box 1159
Sherborn, MA 01770
(888) 440-2963   (508) 651-2963   FAX (508) 650-4216
e-mail: ordering@aquariusproductions.com
www.aquariusproductions.com

This videotape provides information for families caring for children with disabilities or life-threatening illnesses at home. Includes topics such as family relationships, caregiver burnout, respite care, and funding. 34 minutes. Closed captioned. Purchase, $195.00; one day rental, $50.00; one week rental, $100.00; plus $10.00 shipping and handling.

Medical Imaging: Welcome to the Radiology Center
Starbright Foundation
11835 West Olympic Boulevard, Suite 500
Los Angeles, CA 90064
(800) 315-2580   (310) 479-1212   FAX (310) 479-1235
www.starbright.org

This CD-ROM, designed for children ages 6 to 10, provides information about x-rays, MRIs, and CT scans, including preparation and what to expect during the tests. Also recommends coping strategies to use while undergoing the tests. Free

Parenting Children with Special Needs
United Learning
1560 Sherman Avenue, Suite 100
Evanston, IL 60201
(800) 421-2363   (847) 328-6700   FAX (847) 328-6706
e-mail: agc@mcs.net   www.agcmedia.com

This videotape depicts parents' experiences upon learning that their child has a disability, the effects on the family dynamics, the benefits of early intervention, legal requirements, and how to work with health care professionals. 30 minutes. $95.00 plus $3.00 shipping and handling

Parents' Guide: Accessing Parent Groups
by Suzanne Ripley
National Information Center for Children and Youth with Disabilities
PO Box 1492
Washington, DC 20013-1492
(800) 695-0285 (V/TT)   In the Washington, DC area, (202) 884-8200 (V/TT)
FAX (202) 884-8441   e-mail: nichcy@aed.org   www.nichcy.org

Provides guidelines for locating and/or organizing parent groups; describes community services and how to use them; includes a special section for rural families; and makes recommendations for organizing medical, school, and community services records. Free

Plastic Eggs or Something? Cracking Hospital Life
What Am I? Chopped Liver? Communicating with Your Doctor
Starbright Foundation
11835 West Olympic Boulevard, Suite 500
Los Angeles, CA 90064
(800) 315-2580   (310) 479-1212   FAX (310) 479-1235
www.starbright.org

These videotapes are designed for youngsters, ages 10 to 18, who have serious medical conditions, the parents, and the health care professionals who work with them. Free

Spotlight on IVs
Starbright Foundation
11835 West Olympic Boulevard, Suite 500
Los Angeles, CA 90064
(800) 315-2580   (310) 479-1212   FAX (310) 479-1235
www.starbright.org

This CD-ROM uses animation to help children, ages 6 to 10, understand intravenous procedures and equipment. Also offers relaxation techniques. Free

What is a Pediatric Surgeon?
American College of Surgeons
633 North Saint Clair Street
Chicago, IL 60611
(312) 202-5000   FAX (312) 202-5001
e-mail: postmaster@facs.org   www.facs.org

This brochure discusses the qualifications of a pediatric surgeon. Single copy, free.

When Your Child Needs Anesthesia
American Society of Anesthesiologists
520 North Northwest Highway
Park Ridge, IL 60068
(847) 825-5586   FAX (847) 825-1692   e-mail: mail@asahq.org
www.asahq.org

This brochure discusses the administration of anesthesia to children, the types of anesthesia, post-surgical pain control, and what parents should expect. Free

Your Child and Health Care: A "Dollars and Sense" Guide for Families with Special Needs
by Lynn Robinson Rosenfeld
Paul H. Brookes Publishing Company, Baltimore, MD

This book provides practical information about a wide variety of public and private funding sources for medical care for children with disabilities. Includes resource lists and a glossary. Out of print

Your Child in the Hospital: A Practical Guide for Parents
by Nancy Keene and Rachel Prentice
O'Reilly and Associates
101 Morris Street
Sebastopol, CA 95472
(800) 998-9938   (707) 829-0515
e-mail: order@oreilly.com   www.patientcenters.com

This guide for parents discusses strategies for preparing children for outpatient or inpatient hospitalization. Includes resource list. $11.95 plus $4.50 shipping and handling

Chapter 8

SPECIAL ISSUES FACING ELDERS

(Also see Chapter 5 for information about Medicare
and Chapter 6 for information about drugs.)

There are many special issues that arise when older medical consumers have health problems, not the least of which is ageism. Along with the stereotype that elders are no longer capable of making their own decisions, many physicians encourage the myth that health problems are due solely to the patient's age. Many elders hold this same misconception and therefore readily accept their physicians' proclamation that "Nothing can be done" for symptoms that appear in old age. Many elders associate pain, discomfort, debilitation, or decline in intellectual function with aging per se. The notion that illness and disabilities are to be expected as a function of aging deters many individuals from seeking out services. At the same time, research has shown that interventions may increase elders' sense of control, lessening their sense that decline is inevitable with aging and therefore unremediable (Rodin: 1989).

Robert Butler (1997), a well known geriatrician and founding director of the National Institute on Aging, has commented on the need for elders to take a collaborative role in their own health care decisions and has criticized the notion of placing a "case manager" in charge of the situation. According to Butler, older health care consumers should have full access to all available information about their condition as well as access to their own medical charts.

As in any age group or sub-population, the need for information and to participate in decision-making will vary among individuals. However, there is some indication that the current population of elders may desire less participation in the decision-making process than younger individuals. A study by Beisecker (1988) found that, although elders desired as much information about their medical conditions as younger individuals, increasing age was related to beliefs that physicians should have complete authority to make medical decisions. Subjects age 60 or over were more likely than younger subjects to bring a companion with them to doctors' visits, and these companions were likely to make consumerist comments. Although the accompanying person may intend to be an advocate for the medical consumer, often the interaction among the physician, medical consumer, and accompanying person may result in a conflict, with two of the three parties taking sides against the third party.

ELDERS AND THE HEALTH CARE SYSTEM

Elders use the health care system in disproportionately large numbers. Individuals age 65 and over have the highest rate of office visits to physicians (Woodwell: 1997) and the highest rate of hospital stays of any age group (U.S. Bureau of the Census: 1996). In 1999, individuals 75 years old and over made an average of nearly seven visits to physicians (Cherny et al.: 2001).

In many instances, the aggressiveness of the medical profession in its attempts to cure disease does not factor in the effects of elders' frailties on the proposed treatment. Major surgery may indeed be effective in halting the spread of some cancers in elders, but if their hearts are not strong enough, the surgery itself may cause a heart attack and other serious complications. If the elder is mentally alert, he or she should decide whether or not to pursue surgery or other aggressive treatments, with full knowledge of the likely effects on his or her post-treatment functioning. To most elders, losing the ability to function independently is a serious threat to self-esteem. In order to be certain that the elder's wishes are followed, advance directives and living wills should be discussed with family members or others who are in a situation to make decisions if the elder is unable to communicate his or her wishes (see Chapter 5, "MEDICAL BENEFITS AND LEGAL RIGHTS").

Although surgeons may not always take into account the elder's overall condition when recommending surgery, there is evidence to suggest that elders may not receive all the treatment they need when hospitalized. A study found that elders receive fewer hospital resources than younger patients in hospitals, despite similarities in the severity of illness. Less money was spent on elders, and fewer invasive procedures (surgery, dialysis, and heart catheterization) were performed on older patients (Hamel et al.: 1996).

ELDERS AND HEALTH CARE PLANS

Elders must be especially careful in selecting their health care coverage. Although elders are covered by Medicare, it is important that they have private Medigap insurance to cover the charges that Medicare does not cover. Medicare HMOs receive a monthly capitation payment, which is a flat payment from the government for each person enrolled in the plan, no matter how many services are provided. These plans do not charge a premium to the enrollees, since they obtain their payment up front from the government. Because they do not receive additional payments, it is in the plan's financial interest to provide a minimal amount of services. Other HMOs usually charge a lower fee than fee-for-service plans and a small charge or co-pay directly to the enrollee (usually about $5.00 per office visit). These plans may also be enticing to those on a fixed income. However, the motivation to keep costs down may prove detrimental to the health of enrollees. For example, a study by Retchin and his colleagues (1997) found that patients discharged from the hospital to recover from a stroke were more likely to be sent for rehabilitation if they were enrolled in fee-for-service health plans than if they were enrolled in Medicare HMOs. Patients in Medicare HMOs were more likely to be sent to nursing homes.

Some elders enroll in a Medicare HMO because they have received inaccurate information from the plan's representatives and do not fully understand the plan or what they are signing up for (Wilson: 1995). Unsatisfied enrollees may appeal the denial of services, although many of these appeal processes are impractical, as they take too long to help people who are sick and in need of services. Nonetheless, HMOs have internal appeal processes, and regional offices of the Centers for Medicare and Medicaid Services (CMS), formerly the Health Care Financing Administration (HCFA), the federal agency that oversees Medicare and Medicaid, also take complaints.

Judicial appeals are another avenue for unsatisfied enrollees (Wilson: 1995). A lawsuit filed by a group of Medicare beneficiaries claimed that HCFA (now the Centers for Medicare and Medicaid Services) did not require that beneficiaries receive information about denials of health care services and their right to appeal. The beneficiaries prevailed at both the district and appeals court levels. The district court ruled that Medicare HMOs must adhere to specific time requirements for denying services and specified the type of information that must appear in the notification, and how to handle urgent cases. While waiting for the ruling from the appeals court, CMS issued rules regarding these matters (American Association of Retired Persons: 1998). Medicare HMOs are now required to notify enrollees when they deny, reduce, or terminate services or payment for services and to provide written information about how to appeal decisions, including the time frames for each step in the appeals process. The appeals court went even further, requiring that the federal government not renew contracts with HMOs that fail to give participants the reason for denial of services or notification of their right to appeal within five days. Notices must be in a print size large enough for elders to read (Associated Press: 1998). Enrollees are advised to call the Medicare Hotline, (800) 633-4227, for information on their state's Insurance Counseling and Assistance Program.

Elders enrolled in a Medicare HMO may change their coverage to a different plan by giving 30 days notice. If the current plan does not cover a needed service, the elder may seek out a plan that does provide the service or enroll in a fee-for-service plan (Meade: 1997). A study by Families USA (Knox: 1997) found that elders have a high rate of drop-out from Medicare HMOs. The first study of its kind found that the average national drop-out rate was 13 percent, with nearly two-fifths (39%) of the drop-outs returning to fee-for-service care and the remainder switching to another HMO. For-profit HMOs had higher drop out rates than nonprofits.

Elders who wish to complain about the quality of service provided by their Medicare HMO should contact the Peer Review Organization (PRO), a group of health care professionals responsible for monitoring services to Medicare recipients. For example, if you do not agree with your HMO's decision to discharge you from the hospital, you should ask for an immediate review by a PRO. A review will take at least 24 hours; you may stay in the hospital at no charge during the review period (Health Care Financing Administration: 1996).

LONG TERM CARE

The options available for long term care have increased in recent years. In addition to nursing homes and home health services, assisted living facilities and continuing care communities are available to help elders manage medical conditions. The various options have different costs, and some are reimbursed by Medicare or Medicaid and private insurance, while others are not. Each individual and his or her family must determine which option is best for the specific situation. In any case, the credentials of the providers must be investigated thoroughly to avoid neglect or abuse and to ensure that the individual receives the care and attention that he or she needs.

Variables to consider when deciding the type of long term care that is appropriate are the financial assets available, availability of services funded by the government or insurance coverage, severity of the elder's condition, and ability to conduct activities of daily living such as toileting, bathing, and dressing. The availability of long term care facilities, the cost, and assessment of the quality of their services are also crucial factors in deciding where the elder will live.

In 1997, there were approximately 17,000 nursing homes that had 1.6 million current residents and 2.4 million discharges (Gabrel: 2000). Nursing homes are residential facilities that provide care to individuals who are recuperating from an illness or surgery or have a chronic condition or disability and are unable to care for themselves. Many individuals spend short periods in nursing homes to receive rehabilitation for injuries such as fractured hips or following hip replacement surgery. A small percentage of elders move to nursing homes as a permanent residence; however, the large majority of elders remain living independently in their own homes throughout their lives. Nearly a third of all elders live alone, and only 5% live in nursing homes (U.S. Department of Health and Human Services: 1991).

Nursing homes are certified by Medicare and Medicaid, licensed by state departments of health, and accredited by private agencies. State departments of health monitor these agencies as part of their responsibility to the federal government. When elders and their family members are evaluating a nursing home, they should first contact the appropriate state agency and obtain reports on those agencies that seem likely candidates. In addition, guidebooks that rank and evaluate these facilities are available (see "PUBLICATIONS AND TAPES" section below). Each state has a long term care ombudsman that resolves complaints made by residents of these facilities or on their behalf. The ombudsman can provide you with information about legal rights of residents mandated by both federal and state law.

The *Nursing Home Reform Act of 1987* (P.L. 100-203) was passed by Congress in response to the publicity about abuse and neglect of residents in nursing homes. The Act spells out requirements for assessments of residents, planning individual programs of care, and residents' rights, including the right to participate in decisions about their care program and the right to be free of physical and chemical restraints used for discipline or convenience. Residents are guaranteed the right to voice grievances without reprisal and to have access to the state ombudsman. The law also mandates the type of services that must be provided in each facility and requirements for staffing and training.

Elders who live in their own homes and have medical conditions that require daily treatment may receive home health care, sometimes covered by Medicare, Medicaid, or private insurance. In this situation, nurses, physical therapists, and other health care providers visit the elders, monitoring their condition and performing a variety of medical procedures or treatments. Home health aides help with activities of daily living, meal preparation, and household management. Home health care agencies are certified by Medicare and Medicaid and accredited by the Joint Commission on Accreditation of Healthcare Organizations.

Both assisted living facilities and continuing care communities enable elders to maintain their own apartments while guaranteeing that they will receive the assistance that they require. In assisted living facilities, the resident lives in his or her own unit and receives help with activities of daily living and meals. Continuing care communities enter into a contract to provide health care for the remainder of the individual's life; often they have affiliated nursing homes, so that residents may remain on the premises of the facility and maintain their apartments. Because these facilities offer extended health services, even those who are healthy when they enter the community must pay a fee that covers these services. The Continuing Care Accreditation Commission, part of the American Association of Homes and Services for the Aged, accredits continuing care retirement communities throughout the country. It is wise to contact either an elder law attorney or a financial advisor to help decide if the financial arrangements are amenable to your situation.

It is important to check each residential facility carefully, talking to other residents and evaluating the services and physical plants. Obtain a checklist from an organization that accredits these agencies and facilities. Some continuing care communities will offer the elder and a family member a free stay for one night to evaluate the community and taste the food.

It is important to ensure that health care providers in each of these organizations have been licensed and that the quality of their care has been evaluated. Check with the state department that licenses these providers, prepared with a list of questions to assist your investigation. For example:

- Has the agency ever lost its accreditation or licensure?
- How many and what types of complaints have been filed against it?
- Are the personnel used by the agency accredited in their fields?
- Do they have a history of medication errors? Of overmedicating residents?
- Does the state department of health have a report on its most recent assessment of the facility or agency?

LONG TERM CARE INSURANCE

Long term care insurance is designed to help pay for the expenses for prolonged care if an illness or disability limits independent functioning. Long term care usually involves skilled and personal or custodial care provided in various facilities, such as nursing homes, adult day health centers, or in the home. The cost of long term care is usually not covered by Medicare, Medicare supplemental insurance, or major medical health care policies. About 50% of all nursing home expenses are paid for by Medicaid, the joint federal/state health insurance plan for individuals who meet the federal financial criteria. It is not uncommon for individuals to initially pay out of pocket for nursing home care and then to turn to Medicaid once their assets have been depleted to the levels required to meet federal poverty guidelines.

Long term care insurance policies should be carefully examined before purchase. Typical policies cover nursing home and home care services, but the scope of the policies varies dramatically. A fixed daily benefit, or indemnity, is paid for nursing home or home care. Home care is usually reimbursed at a lower rate than nursing home care. Services such as adult day care or respite care may be covered under some policies. Benefits paid by long term care policies usually range between $50.00 and $250.00 per day. Premiums rise as the benefit level rises. Potential purchasers should investigate the average costs of facilities in the local area. The policy should be examined to determine if the coverage is sufficient for the rates charged locally. Inflation protection increases policy benefits so that they rise with the cost of services. The younger the insured is when purchasing the policy, the lower the premium will be, although presumably the insured will be paying premiums for a longer period of time. Insurance companies may require a waiting period before benefits may begin for individuals who have a illness, such as a heart condition. Talking with a financial advisor may be a wise idea.

Although the cost of long term care insurance is high, for some individuals the cost is worth the peace of mind that the policy brings. The *Kennedy-Kassebaum Health Insurance Portability and Accountability Act of 1996* amended the tax code so that 1) benefits received under "qualified" long term care policies are considered medical expenses and excluded from gross income; 2) employer contributions to long term care insurance premiums will be excluded from gross income; 3) out-of-pocket long term care expenses will be deductible to the extent that they exceed 7.5% of adjusted gross income; and 4) self-employed individuals may include the cost of long term care insurance premiums when determining allowable deduction for health insurance expenses. There are annual dollar limits that vary with the age of the insured. Payment for services provided by a spouse or relative is not considered a medical expense unless the provider is a licensed professional.

Unlike Medicare supplemental insurance policies, long term care insurance policies are not standardized. In addition to insurance companies, employers and associations may offer long term care insurance. The National Association of Insurance Commissioners (see "ORGANIZATIONS" section below), composed of state insurance officials, has developed a model policy that some states have adopted. Under this model plan, insurance companies that sell long term care policies must give prospective customers the NAIC's publication "A Shopper's Guide to Long-Term Care Insurance." It is wise to check the financial stability of the company prior to purchasing any insurance in order to feel comfortable that the company will be in business when you need the benefits. Rating agencies such as A.M. Best Company perform financial analyses of insurance companies and publish guides that are available in the reference section of public libraries. Insurance counseling programs are available through state insurance departments and agencies on aging.

ELDERS AND DRUGS

Special attention must be paid to prescription drugs for elders. Because elders often have multiple health conditions, they take multiple drugs. Changes in the kidneys and liver due to aging affect the body's ability to process and eliminate fluids and toxins. Elders' digestive systems may be unable to absorb food and drugs as well as younger people can. Given the specialization of medical care, it is not unusual for one medical specialist to prescribe a medication, not knowing that the patient already takes a medication that will interact with the new prescription to cause an adverse reaction. It is extremely important for elders and their advocates to make sure that they tell their physicians about the drugs they are currently taking prior to starting a new medication. In some instances, the various physicians involved in treating the patient may need to confer in order to develop a coordinated medication plan. The FDA now requires that all drugs submitted for approval be tested on elders as well as the general population.

One common feature of ageism is prescribing too many medications. Elders who take a variety of medications may find that the interaction of the various drugs causes unpleasant side effects, and some may cause what appears to be mental confusion or impairment. Physicians frequently prescribe psychotropic drugs (antianxiety drugs, antidepressants, or sedatives) to older patients, believing that they will quell the patients' anxieties. Often, however, these drugs deprive medical consumers of their mental alertness, which in turn may increase depression.

Elders' attitudes toward pain may affect their willingness to accept medication. A desire to "tough it out" or a fear of addiction may influence their responses to questions about their pain levels.

In 1998, the American Geriatrics Society released clinical practice guidelines for the management of chronic pain in elders. The guidelines include recommendations on the assessment of chronic pain, pharmacologic treatments, and nonpharmacologic strategies, and the obligations of the health care system to provide comfort and pain management (American Geriatrics Society: 1998). Elders who experience chronic pain may wish to consider maintaining a pain diary in which they record pain episodes; intensity; use of medications and their effectiveness; nonpharmacologic interventions such as applying heat or cold, massage, or relaxation techniques; and activities associated with the pain episode. This pain history will help develop a course of treatment.

An elder's sensory losses may affect his or her ability to properly administer medications. If it is difficult to hear oral instructions and to read the tiny print on a pill bottle, the elder is at risk for misusing the medication. Memory loss may account for errors in under- or over-medication. Many of the drugs commonly taken by elders for heart conditions or high blood pressure may cause depression.

SPECIAL INFORMATION FOR CAREGIVERS

Caregiving has become a way of life for a significant number of Americans. As the population ages, more and more individuals have serious health problems, and their spouses and children often become informal caregivers. According to a study (National Alliance for Caregivers: 1997), over 22 million Americans, representing nearly a quarter of all households, have the responsibility of caring for a relative or friend over 50 years old. Nearly three-quarters of the caregivers are women. The conditions necessitating the care cover a wide range including heart disease, cancer, mobility problems, stroke, or those attributed to "aging." Although most of the caregivers assist with activities of daily living, some caregivers assist with medical management and administration of medications.

Caregivers should use the same methods they use in assessing their own medical care to assess the services being provided to the care recipient. Especially in cases when the care recipient is physically or mentally unable to obtain adequate information, the caregiver should be introduced to the health care personnel as the care recipient's advocate (health care agent or proxy), someone who is entitled to receive information and ask questions.

Whenever possible, caregivers should discuss decisions with the care recipient. Unless the care recipient is cognitively impaired, there is no reason that he or she should not be the one who makes the final decision regarding medical care. In cases when the care recipient has a physical disability that precludes researching the topic at hand, the caregiver should discuss the information gleaned from a literature search and evaluations of health care providers and facilities. Sharing information and enabling the care recipient to make his or her own decision is better for all parties concerned; the caregiver will not fear that he or she forced a decision upon the care recipient, who in turn will feel in charge of the situation.

When Congress reauthorized the Older Americans Act in 2001, funding was included for the National Family Caregivers Support program. This program provides caregivers information about services; assistance in locating services; counseling, support groups, and caregiver training; respite care; and supplemental services.

References

American Association of Retired Persons
1998 "If You're Dissatisfied with Your Managed Care Plan" Perspectives in Health and Aging 13:1:10-11

American Geriatrics Society
1998 "The Management of Chronic Pain in Older Adults" Journal of the American Geriatrics Society 46:5:635-651

Associated Press
1998 "New Rights for Medicare Patients Ruled" Boston Globe August 15 A8

Beisecker, Analee E.
1988 "Aging and the Desire for Information and Input in Medical Decisions: Patient Consumerism in Medical Encounters" The Gerontologist 28:3:330-335

Butler, Robert N.
1997 "The Case for Collaborative Care versus Case Management" Aging Today September/October p. 3

Cherny, Donald K. et al.
2001 "National Ambulatory Medical Care Survey: 1999 Summary" Advance Data from Vital and Health Statistics No. 332, July 10 Hyattsville, MD: National Center for Health Statistics

Gabrel, Celia S.
2000 "An Overview of Nursing Home Facilities: Data from the 1997 National Nursing Home Survey" Advance Data from Vital and Health Statistics No. 311, March 1 Hyattsville, MD: National Center for Health Statistics

Hamel, M.B. et al.
1996 "Seriously Ill Hospitalized Adults: Do We Spend Less on Older Patients?" Journal of the American Geriatrics Society 44:9(September):1043-1048

Health Care Financing Administration
1996 Medicare Beneficiary Advisory Bulletin: What Medicare Beneficiaries Need to Know About Health Care Maintenance Organizations Baltimore, MD: Health Care Financing Administration

Knox, Richard A.
1997 "Many Found to Drop Out from Medicare HMOs" Boston Globe December 5

Meade, Karen M.
1997 "Taking the Risk Out of Medicare HMOs" Advance for Directors in Rehabilitation 6:4(April):47-51

National Alliance for Caregivers and American Association of Retired Persons

1997 Family Caregiving in the U.S.: Findings from a National Survey Washington DC: Author

Retchin, Sheldon M. et al.

1997 "Outcomes of Stroke Patients in Medicare Fee for Service and Managed Care" JAMA 278:2(July 9):119-124

Rodin, Judith

1989 "Sense of Control: Potentials for Intervention" Annals of the American Academy of Political and Social Science 503(May):29-42

U.S. Bureau of the Census

1996 Statistical Abstract of the United States Washington DC: U.S. Government Printing Office

U.S. Department of Health and Human Services

1991 Aging in America: Trends and Projections DHHS Publication No. (FCoA) 91-28001

Wilson, Sally Hart

1995 "Medicare Health Maintenance Organizations: Bright Promise, Troubling Reality" Bifocal 16:2(Summer):3-4, 7-9

Woodwell, David A.

1997 "National Ambulatory Medical Care Survey: 1996 Summary" Advance Data from Vital and Health Statistics No. 295 Hyattsville, MD: National Center for Health Statistics

ORGANIZATIONS

Administration on Aging (AoA)
Department of Health and Human Services
330 Independence Avenue, SW
Washington, DC 20201
(202) 401-4541   FAX (202) 260-1012   e-mail: aoainfo@aoa.gov
www.aoa.dhhs.gov

A federal agency that acts as an advocate for elders within the federal government. Administers grants, sponsors research, and prepares and disseminates information related to problems of elders. Provides technical assistance to state and area agencies on aging.

American Association of Homes and Services for the Aged (AAHSA)
2519 Connecticut Avenue, NW
Washington, DC 20008
(800) 675-9253   (202) 783-2242   FAX (202) 783-2255
e-mail: info@aahsa.org   www.aahsa.org

The AAHSA is a national association of nonprofit organizations that provide housing and health care to elders. The Continuing Care Accreditation Commission, part of the AAHSA, accredits continuing care retirement communities throughout the country. The web site offers "Consumer Tips" on subjects such as "Choosing an Assisted Living Facility" and "Finding the Right Nursing Home."

American Association of Retired Persons (AARP)
601 E Street, NW
Washington, DC 20049
(800) 424-3410   (202) 434-2277   www.aarp.org

A membership organization that advocates on behalf of elders. Administers insurance and investment programs and offers a discount pharmacy service. Free catalogue of publications and audio-video programs. Membership, $10.00, includes "AARP News Bulletin" and "Modern Maturity" magazine.

American Bar Association Commission on Legal Problems of the Elderly
740 15th Street, NW
Washington, DC 20005
(202) 662-8690   FAX (202) 662-8698
e-mail: abaelderly@abanet.org   www.abanet.org/elderly

Advocates on behalf of elders in areas such as health care decision-making, housing, elder abuse, public benefits, age discrimination, and guardianship. Free publications list.

American Geriatrics Society (AGS)
350 Fifth Avenue, Suite 801
New York, NY 10118
(800) 677-9944   (212) 308-1414   FAX (212) 832-8646
e-mail: info@americangeriatrics.org
www.americangeriatrics.org

This professional organization for physicians and other health care professionals provides training and research opportunities. Membership, physicians, $215.00; other health care professionals, $195.00. Includes a subscription to the "Journal of the American Geriatrics Society" and the "AGS Newsletter."

Assisted Living Facilities of America (ALFA)
11200 Waples Mill Road, Suite 150
Fairfax, VA 22030
(703) 691-8100   FAX (703) 691-8106   e-mail: info@alfa.org
www.alfa.org

Trade association of assisted living facilities. State by state listing of facilities and checklist for evaluating facilities available on request. Free. Also available on web site.

BenefitsCheckup.org
National Council on Aging

This interactive web site has the user enter information about health conditions, disabilities, income, and assets (entries are held in confidential) and responds with a list of benefits the user is eligible for and the agencies to contact in the user's local area.

Center for Medicare Advocacy
PO Box 350
Willimantic, CT 06226
(800) 262-4414   (860) 456-7790
www.medicareadvocacy.org

This center, staffed by attorneys who specialize in Medicare issues, provides legal assistance and representation as well as self-help materials. Represents clients who want to appeal Medicare decisions, especially the denial of home health care. Services are free to Connecticut residents and provided for a fee to others. Free publications list.

Centers for Medicare and Medicaid Services (CMS)
formerly Health Care Financing Administration (HCFA)
7500 Security Boulevard
Baltimore, MD 21244
(800) 633-4227   (410) 786-3000   www.hcfa.gov
www.medicare.gov

CMS is the federal agency that administers Medicare and Medicaid. Current Medicare regulations are available on the web site, as are many publications, including those about health care plans.

Children of Aging Parents (CAPS)
Woodbourne Office Campus, Suite 302A
1609 Woodbourne Road
Levittown, PA 19057
(800) 227-7294   (215) 945-6900
www.caps4caregivers.org

Helps caregivers find the appropriate care and support for elders as well as for themselves. Sponsors a network of support groups for caregivers. Publishes a variety of training and resource materials for support groups, a national directory of geriatric case managers, and a bimonthly newsletter, "CAPSule." Membership, individuals, $20.00; professionals and organizations, $100.00.

Eldercare Locator
National Association of Area Agencies on Aging (NAAAA)
(800) 677-1116   (202) 296-8130
www.aoa.dhhs.gov/elderpage/locator.html

A nationwide information and referral service that provides callers with the phone number for a local information and referral service, which in turn provides the name of a local agency that can help with their specific needs. Free

ElderCare Online
www.ec-online.net

This web site offers support for caregivers through ElderCare Forum, an interactive message board; chat rooms; articles; and a bimonthly newsletter, "The Caregiver's Beacon," available free online and by e-mail.

ElderNet
1330 Beacon Street, Suite 268
Brookline, MA 02446
(617) 244-1774   www.eldernet.com

Developed by an attorney who specializes in issues that affect elders, this web site provides information and links related to health, housing, finances, laws, and retirement.

Gerontological Society of America (GSA)
1030 15th Street, NW, Suite 250
Washington, DC 20005
(202) 842-1275   e-mail: geron@geron.org   www.geron.org

A multidisciplinary membership organization for professionals with an interest in aging. Sponsors fellowship program in applied gerontology. Membership, $120.00, includes "Journals of Gerontology," "The Gerontologist," and "Gerontology News" (also available free on the web site).

Infoaging.org
American Federation for Aging Research (AFAR)
1414 Avenue of the Americas
New York, NY 10019
(212) 752-2328   FAX (212) 832-2298
e-mail: amfedaging@aol.com   www.infoaging.org

This web site provides information on age-related diseases and conditions.

Joint Commission on Accreditation of Healthcare Organizations (JCAHO)
1 Renaissance Boulevard
Oakbrook Terrace, IL 60181
(630) 792-5000   FAX (630) 792-5005   www.jcaho.org

This organization provides accreditation to health care organizations including hospitals, home care, long term care, and ambulatory care facilities. The health care facilities must pay for the accreditation survey. Criteria used for accreditation evaluations are described on the web site and in JCAHO publications. JCAHO has a consumer information section on its web site, where it is possible to find the accreditation status of specific facilities. Consumers may file complaints about facilities by phoning (800) 994-6610 or e-mailing to complaint@jcaho.org. Consumer publications such as "Helping You Choose The Hospital for You" and "Helping You Choose A Quality Health Plan" are available. Single copy, free. Also available on the web site.

Medicare Health Plan Compare
www.hcfa.gov   www.medicare.gov

Provides access to information about Medicare managed care plans so that consumers may compare costs, premiums, and the types of services provided.

Medigap Compare
www.medicare.gov/mgcompare/home.asp

Information on this web site enables consumers to compare various Medigap health plans.

National Academy of Elder Law Attorneys (NAELA)
1604 North Country Club Road
Tucson, AZ 85716
(520) 881-4005   FAX (520) 325-7925   www.naela.com

A membership organization of attorneys who specialize in legal problems of elders. Publishes "Questions and Answers When Looking for an Elder Law Attorney," $2.25 plus $5.00 shipping and handling. The "NAELA Member Consumer Registry" is available on the web site.

National Alliance for Caregiving (NAC)
4720 Montgomery Lane, Suite 642
Bethesda, MD 20814
(301) 718-8444   FAX (301) 652-7711
www.caregiving.org

An alliance of several national groups concerned with issues of aging, this organization supports research, outreach programs, and a clearinghouse of resources. The AXA Foundation Family Care Resource Connection database, available on the web site, allows family caregivers to search for information on topics such as medical conditions, hands-on caregiving skills, legal and financial information, coping with caregiving, and community resources. Entries are rated for quality and usefulness.

National Association for Home Care (NAHC)
228 7th Street, SE
Washington, DC 20003
(202) 547-7424   FAX (202) 547-3540   www.nahc.org

Trade association of home care and hospice organizations. Consumer education publications include "How to Choose a Home Care Provider," "How to Choose a Home Care Agency," and "Information About Hospice." Single copy, free. Also available on the web site.

National Association of Insurance Commissioners (NAIC)
2301 McGee, Suite 80
Kansas City, MO 64108
(816) 842-3600   FAX (816) 783-8175   e-mail: pubdist@naic.org
www.naic.org

This national organization of state insurance regulators helps protect insurance consumers through public policy development, model laws, regulations and guidelines, and consumer education.

National Association of Professional Geriatric Care Managers
1604 North Country Club Road
Tucson, AZ 85716
(520) 881-8008   FAX (520) 325-7925
www.caremanager.org

An organization of professionals who provide counseling and case management for frail elders and their families. Members help plan for appropriate care and arrange to hire service providers. A national directory of members is available for $15.00. The "Find a Care Manager" database may be searched online.

National Citizens Coalition for Nursing Home Reform (NCCNHR)
1424 16th Street, NW, Suite 202
Washington, DC 20036
(202) 332-2275   FAX (202) 332-2940   www.nccnhr.org

An advocacy group that promotes quality care for individuals in long term care facilities. Membership, nursing/boarding home/assisted living residents, $2.00; persons age 65 and over, $10.00; other individuals, $40.00; citizen groups and long term care ombudsman groups, based on budget size; includes newsletter, "Quality Care Advocate," published eight times a year; nonmember subscription, $45.00. Free publications list.

National Family Caregivers Association (NFCA)
10400 Connecticut Avenue, Suite 500
Kensington, MD 20895
(800) 896-3650   (301) 942-6430   FAX (301) 942-2302
e-mail: info@nfcacares.org   www.nfcacares.org

A membership organization for individuals who provide care for others at any stage of their lives or with any disease or disability. Maintains an information clearinghouse. Membership, family caregivers, $20.00; professionals, $40.00; nonprofit organizations, $50.00; and group medical practices, home health agencies, etc., $100.00. Membership includes quarterly newsletter, "Take Care!" which provides information and resources for family caregivers.

National Federation of Interfaith Volunteer Caregivers (NFIVC)
One West Armour, Suite 202
Kansas City, MO 64111
(800) 350-7438   (816) 931-5442   FAX (816) 931-5202
e-mail: NFIVC@aol.com   www.NFIVC.org

This national membership organization supports the development of interfaith volunteer caregiving programs for individuals who are chronically ill, frail, or alone. Membership, $200.00, includes quarterly newsletter, "NFIVC Caregiver," discounts on publications and conferences, and listing in national directory.

National Institute on Aging (NIA)
National Institutes of Health
Building 31, Room 5C27
Bethesda, MD 20892
(301) 496-1752   www.nih.gov/nia

A federal agency that supports basic and clinical research on a broad range of issues that affect elders. Funds Older Americans Independence Centers, which test interventions to prevent or minimize functional impairments; the Geriatrics Program, which studies topics such as physical frailty, age-related diseases, and disabling conditions; and the Behavioral and Social Research Program that studies the aging process from a social science perspective. Professional and consumer information publications.

Nursing Home Compare
www.medicare.gov/NHCompare

The information on this web site helps consumers compare nursing homes in their areas. Lists nursing home characteristics, nursing staff information, resident characteristics, and results of state inspections.

Nursing Home INFO
N47213 Ellenberger Lane
Eleva, WI 54738
(715) 287-3233   FAX (715) 287-4728
e-mail: nhinfo@nwltd.com   www.nursinghomeinfo.com

This web site provides contact information for more than 17,000 nursing homes as well as a check list for determining the quality of a nursing home, information about residents' rights, and other information pertinent to selecting a nursing home. Provides links to the web sites of member nursing homes.

SeniorNet
121 Second Street, 7th floor
San Francisco, CA 94105
(800) 747-6848   (415) 495-4990   FAX (415) 495-3999
www.seniornet.org

Maintains network of SeniorNet Learning Centers across the U.S. Teaches computer skills to adults over age 50 and manages sites on America OnLine and the world wide web. The "SeniorNet Newsline" is available on the web site.

Well Spouse Foundation
30 East 40th Street, Suite PH
New York, NY 10016
(800) 838-0879   (212) 685-8815   FAX (212) 685-8676
e-mail: wellspouse@aol.com   www.wellspouse.org

A network of support groups that provide emotional support to husbands, wives, and partners of people who are chronically ill. Membership, individuals, $25.00; professionals, $50.00; includes bimonthly newsletter, "Mainstay." Publishes pamphlets discussing "Guilt," "Anger," "Isolation," and "Looking Ahead." $1.50 each; $5.00 per set.

PUBLICATIONS AND TAPES

Ageline
American Association of Retired Persons (AARP)
601 E Street, NW
Washington, DC 20049
(800) 424-3410   (202) 434-2277   www.aarp.org

A bibliographic database that provides citations and abstracts on social, psychological, economic, political, and health issues related to aging. Available through online services and on CD-ROM.

American Geriatrics Society's Complete Guide to Aging and Health
by Mark E. Williams
American Geriatrics Society (AGS)
350 Fifth Avenue, Suite 801
New York, NY 10118
(800) 677-9944   (212) 308-1414   FAX (212) 832-8646
e-mail: info@americangeriatrics.org
www.americangeriatrics.org

A medical reference for elders and caregivers, with information on the aging process, making medical decisions, and strategies for preventing illness. $26.00 plus $5.70 shipping and handling

Beat the Nursing Home Trap: A Consumer's Guide
Nolo Press
by Joseph L. Matthews
950 Parker Street
Berkeley, CA 94710
(800) 728-3555   FAX (800) 645-0895   e-mail: cs@nolo.com
www.nolo.com

This book discusses how to protect your assets, arrange home health care, and evaluate nursing homes. Also includes information on long term care insurance, Medicare, Medicaid, and other benefit programs. $21.95 plus $5.00 shipping and handling. Orders placed on the web site receive a discount.

Best's Company Reports - HMO
A. M. Best Company
Ambest Road
Oldwick, NJ 08858
(908) 439-2200   www.ambest.com

This company ranks insurance companies on their financial stability, their record on claims payments, etc. Reports on individual insurance companies may be ordered by phone, fax, or downloaded from the web site.

By Your Side: Home Care for Older Adults
National Association for Home Care
228 7th Street, SE
Washington, DC 20003
(202) 547-7424   FAX (202) 547-3540   www.nahc.org

This videotape follows three families who are facing the decision to provide care for an elder at home. 37 minutes. $24.95 plus $3.50 shipping and handling

The Caregiver's Guide: Helping Elderly Relatives Cope with Health and Safety Problems
by Caroline Rob and Janet Reynolds
Houghton Mifflin Company
181 Ballardvale Street, PO Box 7050
Wilmington, MA 01887
(800) 225-3362   FAX (800) 634-7568   www.hmco.com

This book covers a wide range of health problems, including cancer, pain, pneumonia, skin diseases, digestive problems, and sleep disorders. $15.00

Caregiving: The Spiritual Journey of Love, Loss and Renewal
by Beth Witrogen McLeod
John Wiley and Sons
1 Wiley Drive
Somerset, NJ 08875
(800) 225-5945   (732) 469-4400   www.wiley.com

This book uses caregiver stories, interviews, and literary references to provide strategies for coping with the stress of caring for loved ones. It discusses topics such as women and caregiving, emotional stresses, end-of-life concerns, and recovery from loss. $14.95

Caring for Yourself While Caring for Others: Survival and Renewal
by Lawrence M. Brammer
Vantage Press
516 West 34th Street
New York, NY 10001
(800) 882-3273   (212) 736-1767   FAX (212) 736-2273
www.vantagepress.com

This book discusses coping and survival strategies and suggests how to face difficult feelings. Provides community resources and reading lists. $14.95 plus $2.50 shipping and handling

Checkup on Health Insurance Choices
Agency for Healthcare Research and Quality Publications Clearinghouse
PO Box 8547
Silver Spring, MD 20907-8547
(800) 358-9295   (888) 586-6340 (TT)   e-mail: info@ahrq.gov
www.ahrq.gov

This brochure describes health, disability, and long term care insurance; provides checklists and worksheet; and defines health insurance terms. Free

Choosing Medical Care in Old Age: What Kind, How Much, When to Stop
by Muriel R. Gillick
Harvard University Press
79 Garden Street
Cambridge, MA 02138
(800) 448-2242   (617) 495-2600   FAX (800) 962-4983
www.hup.harvard.edu

Written by a geriatrician, this book discusses the issues that face elders in making choices for medical care, whether they are frail, robust, terminally ill, or if others must make choices for them. Hardcover, $19.95; softcover, $14.95; plus $4.50 shipping and handling.

The Consumer Guide to Long-Term Care Insurance
Health Insurance Association of America (HIAA)
1201 F Street, NW, Suite 500
Washington, DC 20004
(800) 879-4422   (202) 824-1600
FAX (202) 824-1722   www.hiaa.org

This booklet provides basic information about long term care insurance, along with a worksheet to evaluate policies. Free. Also available on the web site.

The Consumers' Directory of Continuing Care Retirement Communities
American Association of Homes and Services for the Aged Publications
Department 5119
Washington DC 20061-5119
(800) 508-9442   (301) 490-0677   FAX (301) 206-9789
e-mail: info@aahsa.org   www.aahsa.org

This book provides profiles of over 500 retirement communities and information on how to evaluate them. $30.00 plus $3.50 shipping and handling

The Continuing Care Retirement Community: A Guidebook for Consumers
American Association of Homes and Services for the Aged Publications
PO Box 1616
1650 Blue Grass Lakes Highway
Alpharetta, GA 30009
(800) 675-9253   www.aahsa.org

This book describes continuing care retirement community contracts and provides a checklist and financial worksheet. $10.45

dirty details, the days and nights of a well spouse
by Marion Deutsche Cohen
Temple University Press
11030 South Langley Avenue
Chicago, IL 60628
(800) 621-2736   FAX (800) 621-8476
e-mail: kh@press.uchicago.edu   www.press.chicago.edu

A frank, personal account, written by a woman whose husband has multiple sclerosis, this book describes her caregiving experiences. Hardcover, $49.95; softcover, $18.95; plus $4.00 shipping and handling.

Eldercare at Home
by Peter S. Houts and Laurence Z. Rubenstein (eds.)
Foundation for Health in Aging
American Geriatrics Society (AGS)
350 Fifth Avenue, Suite 801
New York, NY 10118
(800) 677-9944   (212) 755-6810
e-mail: info@americangeriatrics.org
www.healthinaging.org/eldercare

This online manual provides information for caregivers on physical problems such as pain, incontinence, and sleep; mental and social problems such as depression, communication, memory loss, and dementia; and managing care, including daily living issues, advance directives, choosing a nursing home, and community resources. Chapters may be downloaded free.

Going Home: Homecare for Adults
Aquarius Health Care Videos
5 Powderhouse Lane
PO Box 1159
Sherborn, MA 01770
(888) 440-2963   (508) 651-2963   FAX (508) 650-4216
e-mail: ordering@aquariusproductions.com
www.aquariusproductions.com

This videotape follows three adults receiving care at home. It covers topics such as family relationships, community resources, independence, and the role of hospice care. 30 minutes. Closed captioned. Purchase, $195.00; one day rental, $50.00; one week rental, $100.00; plus $10.00 shipping and handling.

Home Care: Coping with Change
Terra Nova Films
9848 South Winchester Avenue
Chicago, IL 60643
(800) 779-8491   (773) 881-8491   FAX (773) 881-3368
e-mail: tnf@terranova.org   www.terranova.org

This videotape helps those whose elderly relatives need special health care at home understand the issues that they will face. 27 minutes. Purchase, $89.00; one week rental, $45.00; plus $9.00 shipping and handling.

Home or Nursing Home? Making the Right Choice
by Michael J. Salamon and Gloria Rosenthal
Springer Publishing Company
536 Broadway
New York, NY 10012
(212) 431-4370   FAX (212) 941-7842   springerpub.com

This book enables both families and professional health care providers to make informed decisions about long term care based on research, case studies, and interviews with elders. $26.95 plus $4.75 shipping and handling

How to Choose a Nursing Home
Aquarius Health Care Videos
5 Powderhouse Lane
PO Box 1159
Sherborn, MA 01770
(888) 440-2963   (508) 651-2963   FAX (508) 650-4216
e-mail: ordering@aquariusproductions.com
www.aquariusproductions.com

This videotape suggests questions that families should ask when evaluating a nursing home. Includes a guided tour of a nursing home and reviews financial issues. 31 minutes. $195.00 plus $10.00 shipping and handling

Improving the Quality of Long-Term Care
by Gooloo S. Wunderlich and Peter O. Kohler (eds.)
National Academy Press
2101 Constitution Avenue, NW
Lockbox 285
Washington, DC 20055
(888) 624-8373   (202) 334-3313   FAX (202) 334-2451
e-mail: zjones@nas.edu   www.nap.edu

This book discusses the quality of care and the quality of life in nursing home facilities, home health care, and residential care facilities. $47.95 plus $4.50 shipping and handling. Orders placed on the web site receive a discount.

Journal of the American Geriatrics Society (JAGS)
Blackwell Scientific
350 Main Street
Malden, MA 02148
(888) 661-5800   (781) 388-8250   FAX (781) 388-8270
e-mail: csjournals@blacksci.com   www.blackwellscience.com

Produced by the American Geriatrics Society, this journal provides articles on treatments, health services research, and progress in geriatrics. $185.00

Lifelines: Living Longer, Growing Frail, Taking Heart
by Muriel Gillick
W. W. Norton & Company
800 Keystone Industrial Park
Scranton, PA 18512
(800) 223-2588   (717) 346-2029   FAX (800) 458-6515
www.wwnorton.com

This book describes the challenges faced by four elders who have grown progressively frail. It suggests strategies for prevention of frailty in physical, psychological, cognitive, and social areas. $25.95

National Institute on Aging Publications List
NIA Information Center
PO Box 8057
Gaithersburg, MD 20898-8057
(800) 222-2225   e-mail: niaic@jbs1.com   www.nih.gov/nia/health

Describes the publications that are available from NIA for professionals and the public. Free. Publishes AGE PAGE, a series of fact sheets about a variety of health and safety issues related to aging, such as "Considering Surgery?" "Hospital Hints," and "Who's Who in Health Care." Free. Also available on the web site.

The New Ourselves Growing Older
by Paula B. Doress-Worters and Diana Laskin Siegal
Simon and Schuster
100 Front Street
Riverside, NJ 08075
(888) 866-6631   FAX (800) 943-9831   www.simonsays.com

This book provides information and resources for midlife and older women. Topics include aging, sexuality, disabilities, health care, employment, housing, and finances. $20.00 plus $4.98 shipping and handling

Resources for Elders with Disabilities
Resources for Rehabilitation
33 Bedford Street, Suite 19A
Lexington, MA 02420
(781) 862-6455   FAX (781) 861-7517   e-mail: info@rfr.org
www.rfr.org

This large print resource directory provides information about the services and products that elders with disabilities need to function independently. The book includes information on the diseases that cause common disabilities; the major rehabilitation networks; self-help groups; and legislation that affects people with disabilities. Chapters on hearing loss, vision loss, diabetes, arthritis, osteoporosis, Parkinson's disease, and stroke describe assistive devices, organizations, and publications. $49.95 plus $5.00 shipping and handling (See order form on last page of this book).

Selecting Medicare Supplemental Insurance
American Association of Retired Persons (AARP)
601 E Street, NW
Washington, DC 20049
(800) 424-3410   (202) 434-2277   www.aarp.org

This booklet describes the gaps in Medicare coverage and makes suggestions for purchasing Medigap insurance. Free

A Shopper's Guide to Long-Term Care Insurance
National Association of Insurance Commissioners (NAIC)
2301 McGee, Suite 80
Kansas City, MO 64108
(816) 842-3600   FAX (816) 783-8175   e-mail: pubdist@naic.org
www.naic.org

This booklet provides an overview of long term care insurance, describing the types of policies available, benefits, eligibility requirements, and costs. Includes lists of state insurance departments, agencies on aging, and insurance counseling programs. Two worksheets help consumers evaluate the availability and costs of local long term care and compare policies. $.60

Social Security, Medicare & Pensions
by Joseph Matthews and Dorothy Matthews Berman
Nolo Press
950 Parker Street
Berkeley, CA 94710
(800) 728-3555   FAX (800) 645-0895   e-mail: cs@nolo.com
www.nolo.com

This book discusses eligibility for retirement and medical benefits, your legal rights to Social Security retirement and disability benefits, Medicare, and Medicaid. $24.95 plus $5.00 shipping and handling. Orders placed on the web site receive a discount.

Talking with Your Doctor: A Guide for Older People
National Institute on Aging (NIA)
NIA Information Center
PO Box 8057
Gaithersburg, MD 20898-8057
(800) 222-2225   e-mail: niaic@jbs1.com   www.nih.gov/nia/health

This booklet suggests how elders can take an active role in their health care. Includes tips for choosing a physician, obtaining information, and discussing tests, treatments, and sensitive subjects. Large print. Free. Also available on the web site.

2001 Guide to Health Insurance for People with Medicare: Choosing a Medigap Policy
Centers for Medicare and Medicaid Services (CMS)
formerly Health Care Financing Administration (HCFA)
7500 Security Boulevard
Baltimore, MD 21244
(800) 633-4227   (410) 786-3000   www.hcfa.gov
www.medicare.gov

This book provides basic information on the two parts of Medicare, what Medicare and medigap policies cover, how much medigap policies cost, and your rights to purchase medigap insurance. Available in large print (English and Spanish), audiocassette (English and Spanish), and braille. Free

What Everyone Should Know about Skilled Nursing Facilities Under Medicare
Centers for Medicare and Medicaid Services (CMS)
formerly Health Care Financing Administration (HCFA)
7500 Security Boulevard
Baltimore, MD 21244
(800) 633-4227   (410) 786-3000   www.hcfa.gov
www.medicare.gov

This booklet describes standards, eligibility requirements, and Medicare coverage for skilled nursing facilities. Also lists services not covered. Free. Also available on the web site.

When Your Parent Needs You: Caring for an Aging Parent
Aquarius Health Care Videos
5 Powderhouse Lane
PO Box 1159
Sherborn, MA 01770
(888) 440-2963   (508) 651-2963   FAX (508) 650-4216
e-mail: ordering@aquariusproductions.com
www.aquariusproductions.com

This videotape presents the positive aspects of caregiving. Suggests strategies for dealing with the stresses and life changes. 30 minutes. Purchase, $90.00; one day rental, $50.00; plus $10.00 shipping and handling.

Your Guide to Choosing a Nursing Home
Centers for Medicare and Medicaid Services (CMS)
formerly Health Care Financing Administration (HCFA)
7500 Security Boulevard
Baltimore, MD 21244
(800) 633-4227   (410) 786-3000   www.hcfa.gov
www.medicare.gov

This booklet describes long term care options, discusses factors that affect choice, and makes recommendations for resident care after admission. Free. Also available on the web site.

Chapter 9

PEOPLE WITH CHRONIC ILLNESSES AND DISABILITIES
AND
THE HEALTH CARE SYSTEM

Chronic illnesses often require changes in lifestyle and administration of medications. Individuals with chronic illnesses must take responsibility for their own care, learning what to do during progression or flares of the condition, when it is necessary to see a physician, and when an emergency requires immediate hospitalization. Individuals with a chronic illness must find physicians with whom they can maintain trusting relationships. The overwhelming nature of the time commitment and emotional stress of such illnesses have been described by a psychologist with a chronic illness as follows:

> I find myself increasingly occupied with being a patient, my time taken up with the business of being ill...It takes patience to have to put something off because I'm not up to it today, patience when having a disease gets in the way of having a life...One medical episode flows into another... (Rumpf: 1997).

Individuals with chronic illnesses have indicated that physicians view the diagnosis of such a condition as a dead end, without offering much in the way of support for coping. In Thorne's study (1993), patients complained that their physicians failed to explain the details of their illnesses. Patients complained about insensitive remarks on the part of health professionals, especially the oft repeated statement, "There's nothing that can be done." As patients learned that they could be in charge, they utilized other resources, such as support groups, medical libraries, and other professionals and developed the confidence to make their own decisions.

Chronic illnesses often cause disabilities. For example, multiple sclerosis often causes mobility impairments and visual impairments. Diabetes may cause visual impairments and in some cases, amputation of a lower extremity. Osteoporosis and arthritis both cause mobility impairments. Individuals who have disabilities often must be extremely assertive and resourceful in order to obtain assistance in the form of services and devices that help them maintain a decent quality of life. A number of studies have documented the fact that many physicians fail to refer patients with disabilities for services that may help them remain independent (see, for example, Albert and Helm-Estabrooks: 1988; Greenblatt: 1989).

In many if not most instances, individuals with disabilities must seek out service agencies, helpful devices, and training on their own. A good place to start is the state vocational rehabilitation agency. State vocational rehabilitation agencies provide services directly and contract with private agencies and therapists. After determining a prospective client's eligibility, the vocational rehabilitation counselor will develop an Individual Written Rehabilitation Program jointly with the consumer. Rehabilitation may include rehabilitation counseling; job placement; provision of adaptive equipment, prostheses, and medical supplies; vocational training to remain in one's current position or to learn a new skill; adapting the home or work environment; training in activities of daily living and homemaking; and transportation services.

Just as they must be assertive and determined with the health care system, consumers with disabilities must be vigilant with the rehabilitation system, researching what the government guarantees as their rightful services. The Client Assistance Program is a federally mandated program that requires states to provide information to all clients and potential clients about the benefits available under the Rehabilitation Act and to assist clients in obtaining these benefits.

SELECTING A PHYSICIAN

Individuals with chronic illness or disabilities face a lifetime of visits to physicians and other health care providers for treatment of their medical conditions. They have special needs regarding the physician and the physical facility in which he or she practices. Although the Americans with Disabilities Act mandates that public buildings, including medical offices, be accessible, it is clear that not all facilities have complied. Prior to making an appointment with a new physician, a phone call should be made to ascertain whether the facility is accessible. Specific information regarding the physical adaptations in relation to your special needs should be determined prior to making any appointments. Is handicapped parking available? Is there elevator access to offices located on upper or lower floors? Patients should not be faced with a steep flight of stairs when entering a medical building. Restrooms should be located nearby, and they should have wide doors for easy access for individuals who use walkers or wheelchairs. Physicians who specialize in serving older patients, such as rheumatologists, should ensure that their offices are located near a building entrance so that elders and other individuals with disabilities have only a short distance to walk from the parking lot. Wheelchairs should be available for patients who are frail and cannot walk far. Waiting rooms should have good lighting, comfortable furniture, and current reading material, including information appropriate to the physician's specialty. Alternatively, you may also wish to ask if the physician makes home visits.

Once you have determined that you will be able to enter the building and the specific offices you need to visit, then questions about the physician's practice should follow (see Chapter 2, "Locating Appropriate Medical Care").

Many physicians have limited experience providing services to individuals with disabilities. Crewe (1993) refers to a model type of patient-physician relationship for people with disabilities as a consumer-consultant relationship, with greater equality between the participants. Because people who have lived with the chronic illness or disability for a period of time often become experts not only on the condition itself, but also on their own bodies, they have valuable information to offer to health care providers. Real life experience, however, suggests that the model relationship often does not exist. For example, a report by Binsfeld (1994), a woman who is blind, suggests that physicians discriminate against individuals with disabilities, failing to believe that their symptoms are real and suggesting that instead of physical treatment they obtain psychological treatment. Although physicians often suggest psychological treatment for individuals who do not have chronic illnesses or disabilities, it is likely that physicians hold the same stereotypes about individuals with chronic illnesses or disabilities as other members of society do.

A study of patients' views of their interactions with physicians found that physicians had unrealistic expectations of patients with disabilities. Thorne (1990) found that women with disabilities felt that the health care system did not recognize the impact of their disease on their ability to perform their roles as mothers. Health care professionals expected these women to spend all of their energy managing their disease. The women, in turn, felt inadequate as mothers and that they did not receive proper assistance. Fatigue and mobility impairments precluded their participation in preparing meals and doing housework and made them less consistently available to their children than other mothers. They also feared being overly dependent upon their children.

Gill (1991) observed that traditional medical training focuses on the physical aspects of disability and ignores the social realities of living with a disability. She recommends that physicians and other health professionals go beyond traditional medical training and get to know individuals with disabilities who live and work independently and successfully. This knowledge should enable professionals to refer individuals with recently diagnosed disabilities and their families to other individuals with disabilities; these relationships may contribute to the development or renewal of self-esteem and independence.

In order to assess the capabilities of a medical practice in regard to treating individuals with chronic illnesses or disabilities, inquire about the physician's experiences, as well as the training the office staff has had. Obtaining as much information as possible over the phone can save frustration and unsatisfactory encounters at the office. Ask if the physician is a member of any organizations that focus on disabling conditions, such as the National Multiple Sclerosis Society, the National Spinal Cord Injury Association, or the Epilepsy Foundation. Membership in such organizations suggests a special interest in disability and participation in professional and public education activities.

Once your questions have been answered to your satisfaction, make an appointment that enables you to use any special transportation services that are necessary. Ask how long the appointment will take, and make it clear that a special service will be coming to pick you up, so that you must be finished on time.

When you meet with the physician, a basic interview should make it apparent whether the physician has indeed had experience with individuals who have conditions similar to yours. You should also learn quickly what the physician's attitudes are concerning the ability of individuals with chronic illnesses or disabilities to function independently. It is important that his or her attitudes be compatible with your own. Consider the following when evaluating your visit:

  • Does the physician seem knowledgeable about community
  resources?
  • Does the physician work with a team of health care professionals
  such as physical, occupational, and recreation therapists?
  • Did the physician ask questions about my ability to function at
  work and at home?

Because physicians may have limited experience observing the lives of individuals with chronic illnesses or disabilities and a lack of knowledge about assistive technology and rehabilitation services, they may make recommendations about lifestyles that are inappropriate. A classic result of this phenomenon is that elders who do not hear well are institutionalized for mental problems, because their primary care physicians did not check their hearing and assumed that inappropriate responses to questions were due to mental incompetence.

Even with full knowledge of the condition involved, physicians may make inappropriate recommendations for patients at all stages of life. Irving Kenneth Zola (1991), a prominent sociologist who contracted polio at the age of 16, revealed that his physician, an expert in the care of patients with polio, suggested that Zola live in an institution where he would receive his schooling. The physician believed that Zola would undoubtedly be unable to handle the stairs where his family lived. Zola and his family were determined that he return to his own high school and be back with his old friends, a feat that they accomplished. He reflected upon this decision as follows:

> A lesson from this incident took root. I became skeptical of any authority who made sweeping judgments deemed to be in someone else's best interests... people must be allowed to take certain risks; few, if any, decisions were purely medical. I had the right even at sixteen to choose whether at thirty I might be seriously in-capacitated. This was my first conscious attempt to avoid being invalidated as a person (Zola: 1991, 3).

Just as Zola decided early on that he was going to be responsible for decisions regarding his own fate, many individuals with chronic illnesses or disabilities take the approach that they will be the decision-makers for health issues as well as life issues. Thorne and Robinson (1988) interviewed individuals with chronic illnesses who initially trusted their health care providers, only to learn that the recommendations the professionals made did not take into account the individuals' values. Many of these individuals became experts on the medical aspects of their conditions and sought a relationship with their physicians that was more egalitarian than authoritarian. They sought to impress upon their physicians that they were competent by reading as much as they could about their conditions and trying to establish social contacts with the physicians. The study concluded that when patients are trusted as being competent by their physicians, the patients in turn increase their trust of the physicians.

SELECTING A HEALTH CARE PLAN

It is not unusual for individuals with chronic illnesses and disabilities to require health care that is substantively different and more extensive than individuals who are generally healthy. Therefore, the cost of health care for individuals with chronic conditions and disabilities is likely to be more costly than it is for others. The limitations set by managed care may make this type of health care plan inadequate for individuals with chronic illnesses and disabilities. At the same time, the health care plan choices available are becoming more limited. Many employers are offering choices among various managed care plans, and fee-for-service plans are becoming so expensive that they are out of reach for many Americans. Managed care health plans have often required that consumers select new specialists who are affiliated with the plan, even though the consumers have had their own specialist caring for them for many years.

It is wise to learn about the various services provided as well as restrictions imposed prior to enrolling in a health care plan. Check to be certain that you may select your own physician and that there are physicians on staff who are familiar with your condition. Try to obtain phone interviews with several physicians who are likely candidates. Determine whether enrollees select specialists or if the plan assigns them to specialists. If the plan assigns enrollees to specialists who work for the plan, learn as much as you can about the specialists you are likely to need. Also be certain that the facility is physically accessible (see above).

OTHER SOURCES OF INFORMATION

There are many voluntary organizations dedicated to helping people with specific diseases or conditions cope. The local United Way office or a physician who specializes in the condition should be able to make a referral. Check the Encyclopedia of Associations at the library or other directories of local agencies. Use a search engine on the Internet to find these organizations, as most have their own web sites. The clearinghouses listed in the "ORGANI-ZATIONS" section below are also good sources of information about these organizations.

References

Albert, Martin and Nancy Helm-Estabrooks
1988   "Diagnosis and Treatment of Aphasia, Part II" JAMA 259:8(February 26):1205-1210
Binsfeld, Lisa
1994   "Dealing with the Health-Care System Can Be a Frustrating Experience" Connections
       September p. 6
Crewe, Nancy M.
1993   "Ageing and Severe Physical Disability" pp. 355-361 in Mark Nagler (ed.) Perspectives
       on Disability Palo Alto, CA: Health Markets Research
Gill, Carol J.
1991   "Treating Families Coping with Disability: Doing No Harm" in Rehabilitation Medicine
       Adding Life to Years (Special Issue) The Western Journal of Medicine 154(May):624-
       625
Greenblatt, Susan L.
1989   "The Need for Coordinated Care" pp. 25-38 in Susan L. Greenblatt (ed.) Providing
       Services for People with Vision Loss: A Multidisciplinary Perspective Lexington, MA:
       Resources for Rehabilitation
Rumpf, Terri Pomerantz
1997   "The Business of Being Ill" The Moisture Seekers Newsletter Sjogren's Syndrome
       Foundation September p. 5

Thorne, Sally E.

1993 Negotiating Health Care: The Social Context of Chronic Illness Newbury Park, CA:
Sage

1990 "Mothers with Chronic Illness: A Predicament of Social Construction" Health Care for
Women International 11:209-221

Thorne, Sally E. and Carole A. Robinson

1988 "Reciprocal Trust in Health Care Relationships" Journal of Advanced Nursing 13:782-
789

Zola, Irving Kenneth

1991 "Bringing Our Bodies and Our Selves Back In: Reflections on a Past, Present, and
Future Medical Sociology" Journal of Health and Social Behavior 32(March):1-16

ORGANIZATIONS

American Self-Help Clearinghouse
100 Hanover Avenue, Suite 202
Cedar Knolls, NJ 07927
(973) 326-6789   FAX (973) 326-9467   www.selfhelpgroups.org

Provides information and contacts for national self-help groups, information on model groups and individuals who are starting new networks, and state or local self-help clearinghouses.

Genetic Alliance
4301 Connecticut Avenue, NW, Suite 404
Washington, DC 20008
(800) 336-4363   (202) 966-5557   FAX (202) 966-8553
e-mail: info@geneticalliance.org   www.geneticalliance.org

This coalition of individuals, professionals, and genetic support groups provides education and services to families and individuals affected by genetic disorders. Membership, individuals, $35.00; genetic support groups, $55.00; other organizations, $75.00; includes monthly newsletter, "ALERT." Publishes "Alliance Directory of National Genetic Support Organizations and Related Resources;" members, $15.00; nonmembers, $35.00. Also available as searchable database online.

National Health Information Center (NHIC)
Office of Disease Prevention and Health Promotion
PO Box 1133
Washington, DC 20013-1133
(800) 336-4797   In MD, (301) 565-4167   FAX (301) 984-4256
FAXBACK (301) 468-1204   e-mail: nhicinfo@health.org   nhic-nt.health.org

Maintains a database of health-related organizations and a library. Provides referrals related to health issues for both professionals and consumers. Publications enable individuals to locate information and resources in the federal government. Free publications list.

National Institute on Disability and Rehabilitation Research (NIDRR)
U.S. Department of Education
400 Maryland Avenue, SW
Washington, DC 20202
(202) 205-8134   (202) 205-4475 (TT)   FAX (202) 205-8515
www.ed.gov/offices/OSERS/NIDRR

A federal agency that supports research into various aspects of disability and rehabilitation, including demographic analyses, social science research, and the development of assistive devices.

National Rehabilitation Information Center (NARIC)
1010 Wayne Avenue, Suite 800
Silver Spring, MD 20910
(800) 346-2742   (301) 562-2400   (301) 495-5626 (TT)
FAX (301) 562-2401   e-mail: naric@capaccess.org   www.naric.com

A federally funded center that responds to telephone and mail inquiries about disabilities and support services. Maintains REHABDATA, a database with publications and research references. Some NARIC publications are available on the web site.

National Self-Help Clearinghouse/CUNY
Graduate School and University Center of the City University of New York
365 5th Avenue, Suite 3300
New York, NY 10016
(212) 817-1822   e-mail: info@selfhelpweb.org   www.selfhelpweb.org

Makes referrals to local self-help groups.

Rehabilitation Services Administration (RSA)
U.S. Department of Education
400 Maryland Avenue, SW
Washington, DC 20202
(800) 872-5327   (202) 205-5482   FAX (202) 205-9874
www.ed.gov/offices/OSERS/RSA

Authorized by the Rehabilitation Act of 1973 and its amendments, RSA oversees programs that help individuals with physical or mental disabilities to obtain employment through the provision of counseling, medical and psychological services, job training, and other individualized services. RSA provides funds to state vocational rehabilitation agencies, which in turn provide these services to individuals with disabilities. The Client Assistance Program (CAP) provides information and advice to all applicants for services provided under the Rehabilitation Act of 1973 and its amendments and benefits provided under Title I of the Americans with Disabilities Act of 1990.

Untangling the Web
West Virginia Rehabilitation Research and Training Center
806 Allen Hall, PO Box 6122
Morgantown, WV 26506
(304) 293-5314 (V/TT)   e-mail: walls@rtc1.icdi.wvu.edu
www.icdi.wvu.edu

This web site provides links to a wide variety of other web sites, organized by disability.

Well Spouse Foundation
30 East 40th Street, Suite PH
New York, NY 10016
(800) 838-0879   (212) 685-8815   FAX (212) 685-8676
e-mail: wellspouse@aol.com   www.wellspouse.org

A network of support groups that provide emotional support to husbands, wives, and partners of people who are chronically ill. Membership, individuals, $25.00; professionals, $50.00; includes bimonthly newsletter, "Mainstay." Publishes pamphlets discussing "Guilt," "Anger," "Isolation," and "Looking Ahead." $1.50 each; $5.00 per set.

After the Diagnosis
by JoAnn LeMaistre
Alpine Guild
PO Box 4846
Dillon, CO 80435
(800) 869-9559   FAX (970) 269-9378
e-mail: information@alpineguild.com
www.alpineguild.com

Written by a woman with multiple sclerosis, this book describes the emotional responses to health changes due to physical disabilities, chronic illness, and aging. $12.95 plus $3.00 shipping and handling

Chronic Illness: The Constant Companion
United Learning
1560 Sherman Avenue, Suite 100
Evanston, IL 60201
(800) 421-2363   (847) 328-6700   FAX (847) 328-6706
e-mail: agc@mcs.net   www.agcmedia.com

This videotape relates the stories of individuals who cope with a chronic illness. Includes discussion of changes in lifestyle and relationships as well as emotional issues. 32 minutes $95.00 plus $3.00 shipping and handling

Encyclopedia of Disability and Rehabilitation
by Arthur E. Dell Orto and Robert P. Marinelli (eds.)
Macmillan Library Reference, New York, NY

Written by a variety of experts in the field of disability, this reference book includes articles ranging from AIDS to stroke, advocacy to wheelchairs, and aging to work. Out of print

Mainstay: For the Well Spouse of the Chronically Ill
by Maggie Strong
Bradford Books
45 Lyman Road
Northampton, MA 01060
(413) 586-5207

Written by a woman whose husband was diagnosed with multiple sclerosis at age 46, this book provides her personal account and others' stories, practical suggestions, and advice from health care professionals. $15.00 plus $3.00 shipping and handling; prepayment by check required.

A Man's Guide to Coping with Disability
Resources for Rehabilitation
33 Bedford Street, Suite 19A
Lexington, MA 02420
(781) 862-6455   FAX (781) 861-7517   e-mail: info@rfr.org
www.rfr.org

This book includes information about men's responses to disability, with a special emphasis on the values men place on independence, occupational achievement, and physical activity. Information on finding local services, self-help groups, laws that affect men with disabilities, sports and recreation, and employment is applicable to men with any type of disability or chronic condition.   Chapters on prostate conditions, coronary heart disease, diabetes, HIV/AIDS, multiple sclerosis, spinal cord injury, and stroke include information about the disease or condition, psychological aspects, sexual functioning, where to find services, environmental adaptations, and annotated entries of organizations, publications and tapes, and resources for assistive devices. Includes e-mail addresses and Internet resources. $44.95 plus $5.00 shipping and handling (See last page of this book for order form.)

NORD Resource Guide
National Organization for Rare Disorders (NORD)
100 Rt. 37, PO Box 8923
New Fairfield, CT 06812-8923
(800) 999-6673   (203) 746-6518   (203) 746-6927 (TT)
FAX (203) 746-6481   e-mail: orphan@rarediseases.org
www.rarediseases.org

This directory lists organizations that support individuals with rare diseases and disabilities. $45.00 plus $5.00 shipping and handling

Ragged EDGE
Advocado Press
PO Box 145
Louisville, KY 40201
e-mail: editor@ragged-edge-mag.com
www.ragged-edge-mag.com

This bimonthly magazine reports on disability issues from the perspective of disability rights activists. Individuals, $17.50; institutions, $35.00. Available free online.

Resources for People with Disabilities and Chronic Conditions
Resources for Rehabilitation
33 Bedford Street, Suite 19A
Lexington, MA 02420
(781) 862-6455   FAX (781) 861-7517   e-mail: info@rfr.org
www.rfr.org

This comprehensive resource guide includes chapters on spinal cord injury, low back pain, diabetes, multiple sclerosis, hearing and speech impairments, vision impairment and blindness, and epilepsy. Each chapter includes information about the disease or condition; psychological aspects of the condition; professional service providers; environmental adaptations; assistive devices; and descriptions of organizations, publications, and products. Chapters on rehabilitation services, independent living, self-help, laws that affect people with disabilities (including the ADA), and making everyday living easier. Special information for children is also included. $54.95 plus $8.00 shipping and handling (See order form on last page of this book.)

The Self-Help Sourcebook Online
American Self-Help Clearinghouse
100 Hanover Avenue, Suite 202
Cedar Knolls, NJ 07927
(973) 326-6789   FAX (973) 326-9467   www.selfhelpgroups.org

This online database provides information on national and model self-help groups, online mutual help groups and networks, and self-help clearinghouses. Includes ideas on starting self-help groups and opportunities to link with others to develop new groups.

Unending Work and Care: Managing Chronic Illness at Home
by Juliet M. Corbin and Anselm Strauss
Jossey-Bass Inc., San Francisco, CA

This book analyzes the issues that affect the lives of individuals with chronic illness and their family members. Describes physical and emotional needs; the role of health care personnel; and the means to manage chronic illness effectively. Out of print

A Woman's Guide to Coping with Disability
Resources for Rehabilitation
33 Bedford Street, Suite 19A
Lexington, MA 02420
(781) 862-6455   FAX (781) 861-7517   e-mail: info@rfr.org
www.rfr.org

This book addresses the special needs of women with disabilities and chronic conditions, such as social relationships, sexual functioning, pregnancy, childrearing, caregiving, and employment. Special attention is paid to ways in which women can advocate for their rights with the health care and rehabilitation systems. Written for women in all age categories, the book has chapters on the disabilities that are most prevalent in women or likely to affect the roles and physical functions unique to women. Included are arthritis, diabetes, epilepsy, lupus, multiple sclerosis, osteoporosis, and spinal cord injury. Each chapter also includes information about the condition, service providers, and psychological aspects plus descriptions of organizations, publications and tapes, and special assistive devices. Includes e-mail addresses and Internet resources. $44.95 plus $5.00 shipping and handling (See last page of this book for order form.)

Chapter 10

MAKING DECISIONS ABOUT CURRENT MEDICAL CONTROVERSIES

As new diagnostic procedures and medical treatments are developed, medical consumers must sort out a vast array of information, often contradictory. New treatments, although tested prior to approval for use on humans, still pose risks of unknown dimensions. Drugs may be successful in treating a specific condition, but they may give rise to other conditions. The side effects may develop only after long term usage, so that tests conducted prior to approval did not discover these risks. Virtually every new treatment and some diagnostic techniques are surrounded by controversy.

This chapter discusses some current issues in diagnosis and treatment. Although there are many other controversial medical issues, these are presented as models of how to weigh the risks and benefits of the procedures.

MAMMOGRAPHY

Unlike many other conditions that affect women, breast cancer is one that has received much publicity. Studies about the usefulness of mammography and which treatments for breast cancer are most effective are constantly reported in the mass media, with new studies often contradicting previous studies. Women are forced to sort out the many contradictory findings and recommendations that they learn about virtually every week. Unfortunately, media reports frequently simplify the issues, making it difficult for women to make a wise medical decision based solely on media reports. In general, the media have focused on the age at which mammography should begin and have ignored the interval between mammograms, the number of views of the breast that are exposed, the effect of breast density on the ability of x-rays to detect lesions, the effects of cumulative exposures to radiation, and other imaging procedures that may be more accurate than x-rays.

Reviewing the medical literature on mammography is the only way for a woman to decide if a mammogram makes sense for her, given her age and other related factors. Making a wise medical decision requires a large investment of time, but in the end, women who take the time will feel comfortable that they have all the facts available on this crucial health matter.

Many women undergo mammography because they fear that their risk for breast cancer is high. They have heard that one in eight women will die from breast cancer. This statement is oversimplified. This statistic is not based on actual incidence rates, since there is no national registry of breast cancer cases. The one in eight risk is a lifetime risk, assuming that women live to be 95 years old. Many women and physicians alike are unaware of the conditions under which this statistic was derived; nonetheless, the statistic and its attendant publicity have served to escalate fears among women and caused some women to have mastectomies when in fact their breasts were healthy (Boodman: 1993).

Payer (1992) contends that the "increased" rates of breast cancer are a result of mammography discovering many precancerous lumps, which might have stayed at a precancerous stage throughout a woman's life. Instead, these lesions are detected on a mammogram, removed, and counted as cases of breast cancer.

A controversy surrounding mammography has been about the age at which annual mammograms should start. For several years, there has been a debate about the benefits of mammography for women under age 50. Originally, the American Cancer Society had recommended that all women have a baseline mammogram at age 35, although there was no scientific evidence to support this recommendation (Sox: 1998). In 1993, when the debate over mammography for women ages 40 to 49 heated up, the head of the American Cancer Society counseled women to "ignore the confusion while the experts get their act together" and continue to get annual mammograms (Kong: 1993).

In 1997, a National Institutes of Health Consensus Development Panel recommended that women begin annual mammography at age 50. Citing the lack of research to support the benefit of mammograms for women ages 40 to 49, the panel recommended that women in this age group make up their own minds. Many women's advocates and some politicians contended that this recommendation was based on the government's unwillingness to provide adequate financial coverage for this procedure. Following the vocal protests, NIH reversed its panel's decision, ignoring the scientific evidence the panel had evaluated. Since January 1, 1998, however, Medicare has been paying for annual screening mammograms, without a deductible, for women over age 39 who are covered by Medicare.

The quality of research regarding mammography leaves many unanswered questions. Women who have cancer are more likely to survive when their cancers are caught at an early stage via mammograms than women who do not have mammograms. But how many women exposed to annual mammograms develop cancer as a result of this exposure to radiation compared to women who have not had annual mammograms? This question has not been adequately addressed, although over the years, many experts have believed that the cumulative exposure to x-rays could be life-threatening. The amount of radiation used for mammography has decreased, and the issue is usually not addressed in current literature. However, the National Institutes of Health Consensus Development Statement (1997) reports that the death rate from cancer caused by annual mammograms at the new lower doses could range from none to "much higher than one" per 10,000 women.

Current research has not been able to determine the optimal interval between mammograms. Studies have utilized intervals ranging from 12 to 33 months, and the different intervals showed no difference in reduction of mortality among women aged 50 and over. In women ages 50 to 69, it is thought that lesions remain precancerous for 3.5 years, thus suggesting that screening more frequently than every two years adds no benefit (Kerlikowske et al.: 1995).

The effectiveness of mammography is also questionable because radiologists vary widely in their interpretation of mammograms. When two radiologists who specialize in the interpretation of mammograms read the same set of x-rays, they increase the probability by 8 to 14% that they will discover a tumor that the pathology lab identifies as cancer. However, they also increase their error rate of false positives by 4 to 10 percent, thereby subjecting women to unnecessary surgery (Beam et al.: 1996a). The authors suggest that the wide variability may limit the effectiveness of screening mammography (Beam et al.: 1996b).

Research on mammography frequently uses less than optimal methods. For example, the often cited studies of mammography conducted in Sweden (Nystrom et al.: 1993) compare groups of women who had been "invited" to have mammograms as the experimental group with a control group of women who had not been "invited." However, women who did not accept the invitation and did not have mammograms (ranging from 11 to 26% at five sites) were included with the experimental group in the analysis, and members of the control group who had gotten mammograms on their own were included in the control group. Thus, the results from these studies as well as other randomized control studies were contaminated.

A study (Elmore et al.: 1998) found that nearly half of women had a false positive result after ten mammograms. The authors of this study also state that the rate of false positive mammogram interpretations is higher in the United States than in other countries, suggesting that mammogram interpretation should be studied. Women who receive reports of suspicious findings spend several anxious weeks waiting for the results of a biopsy.

Researchers are now working on methods to replace mammography that will provide immediate analysis of breast lesions. Both magnetic resonance imaging (MRI) and positron emission tomography (PET) are producing promising results (Kaplan: 1997). A study found that MRIs are especially useful for women who have radiologically dense breasts and have compromised mammograms (Harms: 1998). Screening ultrasounds for women who have dense breasts also yielded a higher detection of cancerous lesions than mammography (Kolb et al.: 1998). Digital mammography records x-ray images on a computer screen rather than on film. In 2000, the FDA approved a digital mammography system called the Senographe 2000D (Food and Drug Administration: 2000). Although clinical studies have shown that the method is safe, the evidence to date does not show that this system detects cancer any better than the conventional analog/films. Digital images, however, may be stored and transmitted electronically rather than sending original x-rays for evaluation. They also reduce the need to take additional mammograms because the computer images may be manipulated to allow for under or over-exposure.

As of just a few years ago, only one-fifth of the facilities that perform mammography had received certification from the American College of Radiology (Payer: 1992). The federal Mammography Quality Standards Act (MQSA) of 1992 mandated that as of October, 1994, all operating mammography facilities be certified by the U.S. Food and Drug Administration (FDA). In order for facilities to be certified, they must apply to an accrediting body approved by the FDA, undergo an annual survey by a medical physicist, an annual inspection by a certified federal or state inspector, and meet federal quality assurance standards for personnel, equipment, and record-keeping. The FDA must issue an annual report on MQSA compliance along with a list of the facilities that did not pass inspection. In 1995, the first year that inspections were required, 30% of the 9,510 facilities complied with the new standards. By the following year, of the 2,719 facilities that had been re-inspected, a little more than half had perfect inspections (Food and Drug Administration: 1996). In June 2001, however, 97% of the MQSA-certified mammography facilities were certified (Food and Drug Administration: 2001). States may enact more stringent requirements than the MQSA; facilities in these states must comply with both sets of standards. Veterans Administration facilities are exempt from the regulations of the MQSA. However, they must be accredited by the American College of Radiology and inspected by MQSA inspectors trained by the FDA.

In order to weigh the risks and benefits and to make a wise decision about mammography, women should:

- Review the recent literature to determine which factors are most relevant to their decision (i.e., age, ethnic group, family history, use of estrogen replacement therapy, etc.)
- Obtain recent reports on the safety of mammography equipment and the use of more advanced technology
- Consider genetic testing if they are members of ethnic groups that are susceptible to specific genes that cause breast cancer.
- Discuss the current controversy and research studies with a gynecologist and/or radiologist who specializes in reading mammograms.
- Determine if there are local facilities using more advanced technology for breast screening, such as MRI, PET, etc.

Once a woman has made the decision to have a mammogram, she should seek out a facility that has been accredited by the FDA and displays its FDA Certificate indicating that it meets the MQSA standards. A list of facilities accredited by the FDA is available on their web site at www.fda.gov/cdrh/mammography/certified

References

Beam C.A. et al.
1996a "Effects of Human Variability on Independent Double Reading in Screening " Academic Radiology 3:11(November):891-897
1996b "Variability in the Interpretation of Screening Mammograms by U.S. Radiologists" Archives of Internal Medicine 156:2(January 22):209-213
Boodman, Sandra G.
1993 "The Fear of Breast Cancer" Boston Globe January 6
Elmore, Joanne G. et al.
1998 "Ten-Year Risk of False Positive Screening Mammograms and Clinical Breast Examinations" New England Journal of Medicine 338:16(April 16):1089-1096
Food and Drug Administration
2001 "Facility Certification" MQSA Accomplishments www.fda.gov/mammography
2000 "FDA Approves First Digital Mammography System" FDA Talk Paper January 31, 2000
1996 "Mammography Facility Performance for Calendar Year 1995"
Harms, S.E.
1998 "Breast Magnetic Resonance Imaging" Seminars in Ultrasound CT MRI 19:1(February):104-120

Kaplan, Kathy

1997 "Beyond the Mammogram" <u>National Institutes of Health News & Features</u> Fall pp. 69-70

Kerlikowske, Karla et al.

1995 "Efficacy of Screening Mammography" <u>JAMA</u> 273:2(January 11):149-154

Kolb, Thomas M. et al.

1998 "Occult Cancer in Women with Dense Breasts: Detection with Screening US -- Diagnostic Yield and Tumor Characteristics" <u>Radiology</u> 207:1(April):191-199

Kong, Dolores

1993 "Experts Stand by Early Mammograms" <u>Boston Globe</u> February 27

National Institutes of Health Consensus Development Panel Statement

1997 <u>Breast Cancer Screening for Women Ages 40-40</u> January 21-23, 1997

Nystrom, Lennarth et al.

1993 "Breast Cancer Screening with Mammography: Overview of Swedish Randomised Trials" <u>The Lancet</u> 341:973-978

Payer, Lynne

1992 <u>Disease Mongers: How Doctors, Drug Companies, and Insurers are Making You Feel Sick</u> New York, NY: John Wiley and Sons

Sox, Harold C.

1998 "Benefit and Harm Associated with Screening for Breast Cancer" <u>New England Journal of Medicine</u> 338:16(April 16):1145-1146

ORGANIZATIONS

American College of Radiology (ACR)
1891 Preston White Drive
Reston, VA 20191
(800) 227-5463   www.acr.org
www.radiologyinfo.org

Certifies mammography facilities. An online search may be done for accredited facilities which perform mammography and breast ultrasounds. The web site offers information about mammography procedures, equipment, benefits and risks, and limitations.

Food and Drug Administration (FDA)
Center for Devices and Radiological Health
5600 Fishers Lane
Rockville, MD 20857
(888) 463-6332   e-mail: webmail@oc.fda.gov
www.fda.gov/cdrh/mammography/certified

This federal agency is responsible for regulating the certification of mammography facilities. Its web site has a section called "Mammography Information Service." It is possible to search the web site to determine if a particular facility is certified or to locate a certified facility in your geographic area. The National Cancer Institute can also provide this information at (800) 422-6237.

A Forum for Women's Health
www.womenshealth.org

This web site, created by a woman physician, provides health information by stage of life - girls, reproductive stage, midlife, and maturity. Includes a feature called "Ask a Woman Doctor." Also provides links to other women's health sites on the Internet.

Mammography Help Line
Veterans Administration
(888) 492-7844

Since VA facilities are not certified under the Mammography Quality Standards Act, female veterans should contact the Help Line to obtain information about VA mammography facilities.

Mayo Clinic Women's Health Center
www.mayohealth.org

This web site provides information on health topics relevant to women's health, illness, and sexuality. Offers an online Breast Cancer Decision Guide. Also publishes "Mayo Clinic

Women's Health Source;" $27.00. To subscribe, phone (800) 333-9037; or write Mayo Clinic Women's Health Source, PO Box 56932, Boulder, CO 80321

MEDLINEplus: Mammography
www.nlm.nih.gov/medlineplus/mammography

This web site provides links to general information about this screening procedure, statistics, a directory of FDA certified facilities, research, and resource organizations.

National Alliance of Breast Cancer Organizations (NABCO)
9 East 37th Street, 10th floor
New York, NY 10016
(888) 806-2326   (212) 889-0606   FAX (212) 689-1213
e-mail: nabcoinfo@aol.com   www.nabco.org

This national network of breast cancer organizations provides information to the public and health care professionals. Membership, $50.00, includes quarterly newsletter, "NABCO News" and the "NABCO Breast Cancer Resource List." Ordered separately, the "NABCO Breast Cancer Resource List" is $5.00.

National Breast Cancer Coalition (NBCC)
1707 L Street NW, Suite 1060
Washington, DC 20036
(202) 296-7477   FAX (202) 265-6854   www.natlbcc.org

This grassroots advocacy organization lobbies for funding for breast cancer research and trains individuals as advocates. Membership, $35.00, includes quarterly newsletter, "Call to Action."

National Cancer Data Base
American College of Surgeons
www.facs.org

Reports on oncology outcomes at 1600 hospitals in 50 states. Annotated bibliographies and cancer statistics are also available on the web site.

National Cancer Institute (NCI)
Physician Data Query (PDQ)
CancerNet
CANCERLIT
LiveHelp
31 Center Drive MSC 2580
Building 31, Room 10A03
Bethesda, MD 20892
(800) 422-6237   (800) 332-8615 (TT)   FAX (301) 402-5874
CancerFax (800) 624-2511   e-mail: cancermail@cips.nci.nih.gov
cancer.gov

The National Cancer Institute supports basic and clinical research investigations into the causes, prevention, and cure for cancer. The PDQ database provides up-to-date information on cancer prevention, screening, treatments, and care. PDQ is available on the Internet through CancerNet, which also contains fact sheets and publications, CancerNet news, and CANCERLIT abstracts and citations. CancerFax provides access by fax machine to information statements from the PDQ Database, CANCERLIT citations and abstracts, and fact sheets on cancer topics. Will provide a list of FDA accredited mammography facilities. LiveHelp is a pilot program that provides live, online assistance from an NCI Information Specialist; available Monday-Friday, 12-4 pm, Eastern Time. Most information is also available in Spanish. Calling the "800" phone number listed above connects with the regional center closest to you, which can provide information about the resources described above as well as local resources.

Y-ME
212 West Van Buren Street, Suite 500
Chicago, IL 60607
(800) 221-2141   For Spanish speaking callers, (800) 986-9505
(312) 986-8338   FAX (312) 294-8597
www.y-me.org

Volunteers who have had breast cancer provide information to callers, explaining medical terms and assisting them in formulating questions to ask physicians. Affiliates in 14 states. Membership, $25.00, includes bimonthly newsletter, "Lifeline." Publishes booklets such as "When the Woman You Love Has Breast Cancer," "For Single Women with Breast Cancer," and "I Still Buy Green Bananas: Living with Hope, Living with Breast Cancer." Single copies, free. Some publications are available in Spanish. The web site is accessible in English and Spanish.

Breast Cancer Screening for Women Ages 40-49
National Institutes of Health Consensus Program
PO Box 2577
Kensington, MD 20891
(888) 644-2667   FAX (301) 816-2494
e-mail: consensus_statements@nih.gov
consensus.nih.gov

Published in January 1997, this consensus statement presents both majority and minority statements on the effectiveness of mammography screening for women ages 40-49. Free. Also available on the web site.

FDA Certified Mammography Facilities
Food and Drug Administration (FDA)
Center for Devices and Radiologic Health
5600 Fishers Lane
Rockville, MD 20857
(888) 463-6332   www.fda.gov/cdrh/mammography/certified.html

Updated weekly, this web site lists FDA certified facilities. Individuals may call the National Cancer Institute's Mammography Information Service to locate these facilities; [(800) 422-6237; (800) 332-8615 (TT)].

Harvard Women's Health Watch
PO Box 420068
Palm Coast, FL 32142
(800) 829-5921   e-mail: harvardmed@palmcoastd.com
www.health.harvard.edu/newsletters

Monthly newsletter reports on women's health issues, including conditions affecting the breast and the reproductive system. $24.00

JAMA Women's Health Site
e-mail: WomensHealth@ama-assn.org
www.ama-assn.org/special/womh/newsline

An online service that provides abstracts of articles in JAMA (Journal of the American Medical Association) and other journals that are specific to women's health care concerns.

Mammography and Beyond: Developing Technologies for the Early Detection of Breast Cancer
by the Committee on Technologies for the Early Detection of Breast Cancer
National Academy Press
2101 Constitution Avenue, NW
Lockbox 285
Washington, DC 20055
(888) 624-8373   (202) 334-3313   FAX (202) 334-2451
e-mail: zjones@nas.edu   www.nap.edu

This book reviews and evaluates the current techniques used for screening and diagnosis of breast cancer. It makes recommendations for developing improved techniques as well. $42.95 plus $4.50 shipping and handling. Orders placed on the web site receive a discount.

Mammography Today: Questions and Answers for Patients on Being Informed Consumers
Center for Devices and Radiological Health
Food and Drug Administration
5600 Fishers Lane
Rockville, MD 20857
(888) 463-6332   www.fda.gov/cdrh/mammography

This fact sheet describes the Mammography Quality Standards Act (MQSA) and the rights of women who undergo these exams. Free. Also available on the web site.

Quality Determinants of Mammography: Clinical Practice Guidelines
Agency for Healthcare Research and Quality Publications Clearinghouse
PO Box 8547
Silver Spring, MD 20907-8547
(800) 358-9295   (888) 586-6340 (TT)   e-mail: info@ahrq.gov
www.ahrq.gov

This publication provides an overview for referring health care providers regarding both screening and diagnostic mammography, women with special conditions, such as breast implants, recordkeeping, and communicating the results to patients. Free. Also available on the web site.

<u>Questions and Answers about Screening Mammograms</u>
Cancer Information Center, National Cancer Institute (NCI)
31 Center Drive MSC 2580
Building 31, Room 10A03
Bethesda, MD 20892
(800) 422-6237   (800) 332-8615 (TT)   FAX (301) 402-5874
CancerFax (800) 624-2511   e-mail: cancermail@cips.nci.nih.gov
cancer.gov

This fact sheet explains the difference between screening and diagnostic mammograms, discusses their limitations, and describes other technologies for breast cancer screening under development. Free. Also available on the web site.

HYSTERECTOMY

Hysterectomy (surgical removal of the uterus) is the second most frequently performed surgical procedure in the United States. Although the attention paid to the overuse of this surgery has resulted in a decrease in the number of operations performed, there were still 562,000 hysterectomies performed in the United States in 1993 (U.S. Bureau of the Census: 1996). The United States has the highest rate of hysterectomies of any western country.

By age 60, more than a third of American women have had a hysterectomy. Rates for hysterectomy vary by region of the country, race, and physician gender, with male gynecologists more likely to prescribe hysterectomies (Carlson et al.: 1993). Women with less education and lower income are more likely to have a hysterectomy than women with higher education and income (Kjerulff et al.: 1994).

The most common cause of hysterectomies is the presence of uterine fibroids. Common practice has been to perform a hysterectomy when fibroids cause the uterus to reach the size of a 12 week gestation period, regardless if there are symptoms or not. However, there is no scientific basis for this procedure (Agency for Health Care Policy and Research: 1995). On the other hand, there is no dispute that hysterectomy should be performed when cancer is present. Yet only 11% of all hysterectomies are performed to remove uterine cancer (Agency for Health Care Policy and Research: 1995).

There are several types of hysterectomies: total hysterectomy, which removes the uterus and the cervix; subtotal hysterectomy, which removes the uterus but leaves the cervix; and radical hysterectomy, which removes the uterus, cervix, fallopian tubes, and ovaries along with the nodes and ligaments that hold the uterus in place. Hysterectomies may be performed through the abdomen, through the vagina, or through the vagina with the assistance of a laparoscope inserted into the abdomen.

A quarter to a half of women who have had hysterectomies have post-surgical complications, including abdominal bleeding, blood clots in the lung, damage to the bowel or bladder, and urinary problems (Dennerstein et al.: 1995). Post-surgical recovery appears to be quickest for women who have vaginal hysterectomies, followed by those with laparoscopic assisted vaginal hysterectomies (van den Eeden et al.: 1998). Although many women report an improvement in their symptoms, others have new symptoms that they did not have prior to the surgery. Some women, albeit a minority, report sexual dysfunction following hysterectomy (Dennerstein et al.: 1995).

Alternatives to hysterectomy include more conservative types of surgery, pharmaceutical treatment, or watchful waiting. The decision regarding what type of treatment to have, if any, depends on the woman's condition, her lifestyle and stage of life, her values, and her psychological needs.

Common conditions that result in hysterectomy are uterine fibroids and endometriosis, followed by uterine prolapse, dysfunctional uterine bleeding, chronic pelvic pain, and pelvic inflammatory disease. Uterine fibroids are abnormal growths of uterine muscle found in the uterine cavity or wall or outside the uterine wall. For most women, they never cause a problem, but they sometimes cause heavy menstrual bleeding, which may result in anemia and painful menstrual periods. For these women, gynecologists often recommend either hysterectomy or myomectomy, the excision of the fibroids. Myomectomy may be performed through the traditional abdominal incision. Two techniques for myomectomy have been introduced. Laparoscopy is a procedure in which several incisions are made in the abdomen and a thin fiberoptic tube is inserted, so that the physician may view the abdomen and pelvis. Myomectomy may also be performed using hysteroscopy, a procedure that involves inserting a lighted tube into the uterus via the vagina and cervix. The abdominal myomectomy results in a longer recovery period and more pain than the other procedures.

Both myomectomy and hysterectomy have problems associated with them. Women who have hysterectomies often experience menopause shortly after the surgery. This is especially likely when the ovaries are removed along with the uterus, but even when the ovaries are left intact, they often fail to function after the surgery. Since the ovaries are the source of estrogen, when they are removed or fail to produce sufficient estrogen, women undergo menopause. Decreased estrogen production increases a woman's risk for heart disease and osteoporosis. Myomectomy, on the other hand, removes the fibroids, but they frequently grow back. In addition, the surgery may cause severe bleeding, requiring transfusions. Therefore, the severity of the symptoms and the likely time until natural menopause may determine whether women should undergo either hysterectomy or myomectomy.

A new method to help women with uterine fibroids who experience excessive bleeding during menstruation is thermal balloon therapy. In this procedure, a heated balloon is filled with saline and left in the uterus for about ten minutes. Several studies have found that this method successfully reduces blood flow and eliminates the need for hysterectomy in most women (Barrow: 1999; Ulmsten et al.: 2001).

Pharmaceutical treatments also have their shortcomings. Treatment with gonadotropin releasing hormones (GnRH) is often recommended when fibroids are large. The GnRH reduces the size of the fibroids in order to make myomectomy feasible. GnRH analogs reduce estrogen production and cause a temporary menopause, along with possible hot flashes, headaches, and vaginal dryness. GnRH may only be used for a maximum of six months. Longer use results in increased risk of heart disease and osteoporosis. When the treatment is stopped, the fibroids will once again increase. GnRH agonists help to reduce the negative effects of GnRH analogs, restoring estrogen and enabling longer term use of GnRH analogs (Strausz: 1993).

Watchful waiting is an option available to women with uterine fibroids whose symptoms are not severe and who are approaching the age of menopause. Because fibroids feed on estrogen and menopause results in a decreased production of estrogen, fibroids usually shrink after menopause. Women who experience anemia due to heavy menstrual flow may be helped by taking iron pills. Those who experience severe menstrual pain may take antiprostaglandins in the form of nonsteroidal anti-inflammatory drugs, such as naprosyn.

A study (Carlson et al.: 1994) found that hysterectomy was an effective remedy for uterine fibroids, abnormal bleeding, and chronic pelvic pain. Nearly a quarter of the women in the study who had previously had medical treatment or watchful waiting opted for hysterectomies within one year. This study found more benefits and fewer complications of hysterectomy than previous studies. It has been suggested that the selection method of the participants may have introduced a bias into the study; gynecologists in Maine selected patients for referral to the study (Dennerstein et al.: 1995).

Endometriosis is the abnormal growth of tissue that resembles the endometrium (the lining of the uterus) in other parts of the pelvis, including the ovaries and fallopian tubes, the bladder, bowel, area between the rectum and the vagina, and less frequently, in distant parts of the body (Dennerstein et al.: 1995). Endometriosis is the source of pain when these abnormal tissues bleed during menstruation, and the blood cannot escape. Bending, stretching, exercising, and even standing may be painful. Other symptoms may include infertility, inflammation, adhesions (organs adhering to each other), and bowel problems. The symptoms of endometriosis may continue even after menopause.

Endometriosis is usually diagnosed through laparoscopy. Abnormal tissue and tissue for biopsy may also be removed during this procedure. Treatments for endometriosis include pain medication, hormone treatment with gonadotropin releasing hormones (GnRH), endometrial ablation, or hysterectomy. Endometrial ablation is the removal of the abnormal tissue, which may be done via laparoscopy or hysteroscopy. A laser, electrically heated wire, or heated roller ball is used to remove the abnormal tissue. Hysteroscopy causes menstrual-like pain, dizziness, nausea, and vomiting in a large proportion of women. Ablation is a less invasive and less costly procedure than hysterectomy with fewer complications and a shorter recovery time, but it is not always successful (Dennerstein et al.: 1995). Hysterectomy may be recommended in severe cases of endometriosis; in addition to the uterus, all abnormal growth of endometrial tissue is removed.

In order to make a wise decision about whether to have a hysterectomy or another type of surgery, women should consider the following:

- If more than one treatment option is available, why has my physician recommended a specific option? What are the benefits of this option over the others or watchful waiting? What are the success rates of the various treatments in circumstances that are similar to mine? What are the usual risks and complications that may occur?
- Have new treatments been developed for my condition? If so, how do they compare to traditional treatments in terms of effectiveness and complications?
- What are my risks for heart disease and osteoporosis? Am I better off increasing my risks for these diseases by decreasing my estrogen production or are the symptoms I am currently having less harmful than those diseases?
- Is the research conclusive on the benefits of various treatments in cases such as mine? Are the research methods sound? Do they leave questions unanswered about the effectiveness of the procedures?
- What are the likely effects of the treatment on my sexual functioning?
- If I decide to have a hysterectomy, should it be a total, subtotal, or radical hysterectomy? Which surgical method should be used and why?

• Has the physician suggested a myomectomy, even though my fibroids have not caused any symptoms? If so, what are the reasons for the surgery? What are the risks? What are the benefits?

• Has the physician suggested that I consider hysterectomy even though I am asymptomatic? Are there any indications that I have cancer of the uterus? If not, why did the physician suggest the surgery? A hysterectomy to prevent cancer should be avoided.

• How does my age fit into the treatment decision? Will the loss of my uterus interfere with my plans for having children? Interfere with my self-image as a woman? Decrease my enjoyment of sex? Am I close enough to menopause that my condition will improve when my estrogen production decreases? Am I able to cope with the condition until menopause occurs (at an unpredictable time)?

• What do other women who have had hysterectomies and other treatments for the same condition as I have say about their post-surgical experiences? What symptoms have they experienced, and how would I handle similar symptoms?

Making a wise medical decision regarding treatment for diseases of the reproductive system is crucial to a woman's perception of her body image and her role in society. She must take cultural factors into account as well as the effects of treatment on her relationship with current or future sexual partners. If the woman currently has a sexual partner, the partner should be involved in the decision-making process.

References

Agency for Health Care Policy and Research
1995 Treatment of Common Non-Cancerous Uterine Conditions: Issues for Research
Barrow, C.
1999 "Balloon Endometrial Ablation as a Safe Alternative to Hysterectomy" AORN Journal 70:1(July):80, 83-86, 89-90
Carlson, K.J. et al.
1993 "Indications for Hysterectomy" New England Journal of Medicine 328(12):856-860
Carlson, K.J., B.A. Miller, and F.J. Fowler
1994 "The Maine Women's Health Study: Outcomes of Nonsurgical Management of Leiomyomas, Abnormal Bleeding, and Chronic Pelvic Pain" Obstetrics and Gynecology 83:4(April):566-572
Dennerstein, Lorraine et al.
1995 Hysterectomy: New Options and Advances Melbourne, Australia: Oxford University Press
Kjerulff, K., P. Langenberg, and G. Guzinski
1994 "The Socioeconomic Correlates of Hysterectomies in the United States" American Journal of Public Health 83:1(January):106-108

Strausz, Ivan K.

1993 You Don't Need a Hysterectomy Reading, MA: Addison-Wesley Publishing Co.

Ulmsten, U. et al.

2001 "The Safety and Efficacy of MenoTreat, a New Balloon Device for Thermal Endometrial Ablation" Acta Obstetricia et Gynecologica Scandinavica 80:1(January):52-
57

U.S. Bureau of the Census

1996 Statistical Abstract of the United States 1996 Washington DC: U.S. Government
Printing Office

van den Eeden, S.K. et al.

1998 "Quality of Life, Health Care Utilization, and Costs Among Women Undergoing
Hysterectomy in a Managed-Care Setting" American Journal of Obstetrics and
Gynecology 178:1(January, Part 1):91-100

ORGANIZATIONS

American Association of Gynecological Laparoscopists (AAGL)
13021 East Florence Avenue
Santa Fe Springs, CA 90670
(800) 554-2245   (562) 946-8774   FAX (562) 946-0073
e-mail: information@aagl.net   www.aagl.com

A professional society of gynecologists who perform laparoscopies, this organization will send women a list of their members in order to obtain a referral. Offers a Patients Forum online discussion group.

American College of Obstetricians and Gynecologists (ACOG)
409 12th Street, SW
PO Box 96920
Washington, DC 20090-6920
(800) 762-2264   FAX (202) 863-4994
e-mail: resources@acog.org   www.acog.org

A professional society of obstetricians and gynecologist, ACOG produces professional journals and publications as well as patient education materials. It is possible to search the web site by topic and learn about relevant patient education materials. ACOG will mail five patient education publications at no charge. The Table of Contents for recent issues of "Obstetrics and Gynecology" is available on the web site.

Endometriosis Association (EA)
8585 North 76th Place
Milwaukee, WI 53223
(800) 992-3636   (414) 355-2200   FAX (414) 355-6065
e-mail: endo@endometriosisassn.org
www.endometriosisassn.org

An organization that provides support and information to women and girls with endometriosis. Educates the public and the medical community and promotes research related to en-dometriosis. Membership, $35.00 for women with endometriosis; $40.00 for individuals without endometriosis, physicians, and institutions; includes newsletter, support groups, physician registry list, and discount drug program.

A Forum for Women's Health
www.womenshealth.org

This web site, created by a woman physician, provides health information by stage of life - girls, reproductive stage, midlife, and maturity. Includes a feature called "Ask a Woman Doctor." Also provides links to other women's health sites on the Internet.

HERS Foundation (Hysterectomy Educational Resources and Services Foundation)
422 Bryn Mawr Avenue
Bala Cynwyd, PA 19004
(888) 750-4377   (610) 667-7757   FAX (610) 667-8096
e-mail: HERSFdn@aol.com   ccon.com/hers

Provides information about hysterectomy and alternatives through telephone counseling, referrals to gynecologists, networking with women who have had hysterectomies, and lending library for books and tapes. Publications on a wide variety of topics related to diseases of the reproductive organs and common treatments. Quarterly "HERS Newsletter," $20.00. Free publications list.

Mayo Clinic Women's Health Center
www.mayohealth.org

This web site provides information on health topics relevant to women's health, illness, and sexuality. Also publishes "Mayo Clinic Women's Health Source," $27.00. To subscribe, phone (800) 333-9037, or write Mayo Clinic Women's Health Source, PO Box 56932, Boulder, CO 80321

MEDLINEplus: Hysterectomy
www.nlm.nih.gov/medlineplus/hysterectomy

This web site provides links to general information about the condition, pictures and diagrams, statistics, and resource organizations. An interactive tutorial about hysterectomy is available at www.nlm.nihgov/medlineplus/tutorials/hysterectomy.

National Women's Health Network
514 10th Street, NW, Suite 400
Washington, DC 20004
(202) 347-1140   FAX (202) 347-1168
www.womenshealthnetwork.org

A coalition of consumers, health care providers, and researchers who work to provide up-to-date information about women's health issues and to improve women's ability to make informed decisions about their health care. Maintains a clearinghouse to provide information on a wide variety of disorders and conditions that affect women. Membership, $25.00, includes bimonthly newsletter "Network News."

National Women's Health Resource Center
120 Albany Street, Suite 820
New Brunswick, NJ 08901
(877) 986-9472   FAX (732) 249-4671   healthywomen.org

Develops programs and clinical services to meet women's health needs; sponsors conferences; and provides information to encourage women to be active participants in their own health care decisions. Maintains a database on women's health issues and provides responses to telephone inquiries about specific health issues with referrals, resources, and general information. Membership, individuals, $30.00; organizations, $80.00; includes bimonthly newsletter, "National Women's Health Report."

Obgyn.net
5707 Lakemoore, Suite 100
Austin, TX 78731
(512) 418-2922   FAX (512) 795-0527
e-mail: info@obgyn.net   www.obgyn.net

Developed by health care professionals, this web site is designed for both obstetrician/gynecologists and women who want information about health conditions that are specific to the reproductive system. The site provides up-to-date information about new medical findings, a calendar of events, and a chat room.

Office of Research on Women's Health (ORWH)
National Institutes of Health (NIH)
1 Center Drive, Room 201
Bethesda, MD 20892
(301) 402-1770   FAX (301) 402-1798
www4.od.nih.gov/orwh

Established in 1990, this organization monitors NIH policy with the goal of promoting research into diseases that are prevalent in women, affect only women, have different effects on women than on men, or have different risk factors or interventions for women. ORWH works to ensure that women are represented in NIH sponsored research and to develop opportunities for recruitment, retention, and advancement of women in biomedical careers. Coordinates the Women's Health Initiative (WHI), a research project that sponsors clinical trials, observational studies, and community prevention strategies.

YourSurgery.com
yoursurgery.com

This multimedia site uses simple diagrams and animation to show how a hysterectomy is performed. Click on "abdomen," then on "hysterectomy."

PUBLICATIONS

About D & C for Uterine Bleeding Problems
About Hysterectomy
About Hysteroscopy
American College of Surgeons
633 North Saint Clare Street
Chicago, IL 60611
(312) 202-5000   FAX (312) 202-5001
e-mail: postmaster@facs.org   www.facs.org

These brochures provide information about conditions and procedures that affect a woman's reproductive system. Free. Also available on the web site.

Common Uterine Conditions: Options for Treatment
Agency for Healthcare Research and Quality Publications Clearinghouse
PO Box 8547
Silver Spring, MD 20907
(800) 358-9295   (888) 586-6340 (TT)   e-mail: info@ahrq.gov
www.ahrq.gov

This booklet describes conditions that affect a woman's reproductive system including endometriosis and fibroids and treatments such as hysterectomy. Available in English and Spanish. Free. Also available on the web site.

The Endometriosis Sourcebook
Endometriosis Association (EA)
8585 North 76th Place
Milwaukee, WI 53223
(800) 992-3636   (414) 355-2200   FAX (414) 355-6065
e-mail: endo@endometriosisassn.org
www.endometriosisassn.org

This book discusses treatment options and coping strategies for women with endometriosis along with personal accounts of how the disease has affected women's lives. $14.95 plus $1.95 shipping and handling

Harvard Women's Health Watch
PO Box 420068
Palm Coast, FL 32142
(800) 829-5921   e-mail: harvardmed@palmcoastd.com
www.health.harvard.edu/newsletters

This monthly newsletter reports on women's health issues, including conditions affecting the breast and the reproductive system. $24.00

JAMA Women's Health Site
e-mail: WomensHealth@ama-assn.org
www.ama-assn.org/special/womh/newsline

An online service that provides abstracts of articles in JAMA (Journal of the American Medical Association) and other journals that are specific to women's health care concerns.

The No-Hysterectomy Option
by Herbert A. Goldfarb with Judith Greif
John Wiley and Sons
1 Wiley Drive
Somerset, NJ 08875
(800) 225-5945   (732) 469-4400   www.wiley.com

Written by a gynecologist and a nurse, this book discusses when a hysterectomy is necessary and the numerous situations when it may be avoided. $15.95

Our Bodies, Our Selves for the New Century
by The Boston Women's Health Book Collective
Simon and Schuster
100 Front Street
Riverside, NJ 08075
(888) 866-6631   FAX (800) 943-9831   www.simonsays.com

Written by a group of women, this book provides information on a wide variety of health topics, including interactions with physicians and other members of the health care system and special conditions that affect women. The book includes a great deal of advice about obtaining legal rights within the health care system. $24.00 plus $4.98 shipping and handling

The Real Risks of Hysterectomy and Oophorectomy: What the Doctors Know - and Don't Tell You
HERS Foundation (Hysterectomy Educational Resources and Services Foundation)
422 Bryn Mawr Avenue
Bala Cynwyd, PA 19004
(888) 750-4377   (610) 667-7757   FAX (610) 667-8096
e-mail: HERSFdn@aol.com   ccon.com/hers

An issue of the "HERS Newsletter," this publication includes a review of medical literature regarding the two procedures. $6.00

Understanding Hysterectomy
American College of Obstetricians and Gynecologists (ACOG)
Resource Center
409 12th Street, SW
Washington, DC 20024
(202) 863-2518   FAX (202) 863-4994
e-mail: resources@acog.org   www.acog.org

This brochure describes the uterus and the major conditions that may affect it as well as the different types of surgical hysterectomies and their effects. Free

Uterine Fibroids
American College of Obstetricians and Gynecologists (ACOG)
Resource Center
409 12th Street, SW
Washington, DC 20024
(202) 863-2518   FAX (202) 863-4994
e-mail: mgraves@acog.org   www.acog.org

This brochure describes types of fibroids and available treatments. Free

Women and Their Doctors
by John M. Smith
Grove/Atlantic

Written by a gynecologist, this book discusses the abuse of women by the medical system, medical problems experienced by women, when certain procedures are appropriate, and how to select the right gynecologist. Out of print.

You Don't Need a Hysterectomy
by Ivan K. Strausz
Addison-Wesley Publishing Company, Reading, MA

Written by a gynecologist, this book discusses alternatives to hysterectomy for common problems of the reproductive organs. Out of print.

PROSTATE CANCER

Prostate cancer is the most common cancer in men in the United States and the second leading cause of cancer deaths in men (American Cancer Society: 1995a). The National Cancer Institute (1995) estimated that in 1995 nearly 250,000 men would be diagnosed with prostate cancer and that about 40,000 would die from it. The greatest risk factor for prostate cancer is age; nearly 80% of men with prostate cancer are over the age of 65. African-American men are at highest risk, followed by men who have a father or brother with prostate cancer.

Screening for Prostate Cancer

There is a great deal of controversy over the usefulness of the diagnostic tests now available to detect the presence of prostate cancer. Despite the current lack of evidence that early prostate cancer detection has a net benefit or harm (Barry: 2001), two national health organizations are vigorously promoting screening programs. The American Cancer Society (1995b) recommends that a prostate-specific antigen (PSA) blood test be performed for men annually after the age of 50 and after age 40 for African-American men and men with a family history of prostate cancer. The American Urological Association agrees, recommending that men over age 50 have an annual prostate examination, which includes a digital rectal examination and a prostate-specific antigen (PSA) blood test (Prostate Health Council: 1998). The American College of Physicians, however, recommends that its members inform men about the benefits and risks of screening, diagnosis, and treatment; listen to the individual's concerns; and make joint decisions on whether to screen or not (Rose: 1997). The Centers for Disease Control and Prevention (CDC) concur, indicating that the effectiveness of screening and treatment are not yet known (CDC: 2001). Only a quarter of the primary care physicians surveyed in 1995 conducted PSA testing as a part of routine care only about half the time (Collins et al.: 1997). Effective in 2000, Medicare's decision to approve payment for most of the cost of prostate cancer screening (digital rectal examinations and a PSA test) for all men with Medicare coverage age 50 or over further confuses the decision.

Although it is normal to find small amounts of PSA in the blood, levels tend to rise in men over age 60. False negative and false positive PSA tests have led to questions about the reliability of PSA testing as a tool to detect curable prostate cancer (Prostate Health Council: 1998). Conditions other than prostate cancer may cause a rise in the PSA level. Both prostatitis and benign prostatic hyperplasia (BPH) can raise the PSA two or three times the normal rate (American Cancer Society: 1995b). It may take several weeks following surgery for benign prostatic hyperplasia for PSA levels to return to normal. Finasteride (Proscar), a drug used in the treatment of benign prostatic hyperplasia, lowers PSA levels. Therefore, PSA testing in men who have used finasteride may not be helpful in detecting prostate cancer (Prostate Health Council: 1998). Although there is no benchmark PSA level that indicates a positive cancer diagnosis, an elevation in PSA level can point to the presence of a tumor. Unfortunately, high or low levels can be misleading. If an initial PSA test is positive, it is wise to have the test repeated, in combination with a digital rectal examination. In the American Cancer Society's National Prostate Cancer Detection Project, about 30% of the cancer diagnoses were made in men whose PSA score level was lower than "normal" range; their cancer was diagnosed because digital rectal and ultrasound examinations were conducted in addition to the PSA test (Mettlin: 1997).

In one study, men who were considering PSA screening viewed a videotape that discussed PSA screening, its uncertainties, treatment for prostate cancer, and treatment complications. The men who viewed the videotape were less likely to proceed with PSA testing than men who had not viewed the videotape (Flood et al.: 1996).

The editors of JAMA (Journal of the American Medical Association) questioned the use of the PSA:

> Because many of the tumors detected by PSA would never become apparent clinically, it is not clear that the costs of detection and treatment, and the unpleasant adverse effects of treatment, are balanced by real benefit to the patient (Chabner et al.: 1997, p. 1475)

At its annual meeting in June, 2000, the American Medical Association adopted the following statement:

> The launching of mass screening programs for the early detection of prostate cancer is premature at this time (American Medical Association: 2000)

The AMA policy supports the provision of information to patients about the risks of prostate cancer and the potential benefits and harms of prostate cancer screening. The man who receives this information and who chooses screening should receive both the PSA test and digital rectal examination (DRE).

In a digital rectal examination (DRE), the physician examines the prostate by inserting a gloved and lubricated finger into the rectum. The physician can determine by touch whether the prostate is enlarged or if there are any irregularities in texture. The DRE is used to detect two prostate conditions, benign prostatic hyperplasia, an enlargement of the prostate, and prostate cancer. Although benign prostatic hyperplasia is not cancer, individuals may have both benign prostatic hyperplasia and prostate cancer.

A transrectal ultrasound (TRUS) enables the physician to visualize the entire prostate. A probe, inserted into the rectum, transmits sound waves that bounce off the prostate and create a picture of it on a computer screen. The ultrasound procedure guides a needle that is used to remove prostatic tissue for biopsy (transrectal needle biopsy). The needle may be inserted through the rectum into the prostate or into the perineum, the area between the scrotum and the anus. A biopsy is the only test that positively confirms the diagnosis of prostate cancer. At the same time, a biopsy may give a false negative result if the sample is taken from an area where cancer is not present.

After the Diagnosis

After a diagnosis of cancer is made, the physician will use a staging system to determine the site and location of the disease. This information is used in planning treatment. Stage A is the term used to describe symptomless prostate cancer found during surgery, usually for benign prostatic hyperplasia. These tumors are so small or located so deep in the prostate that they are not found in a digital rectal exam. A firm or hard area confined to the prostate but large enough to be felt during a rectal examination is called stage B. In stage C, the tumor has spread throughout the prostate and into the seminal vesicles, which are located just behind the bladder. In Stage D, cancer has spread (metastasized) to the lymph nodes and other parts of the body such as the bones, lungs, or liver (National Cancer Institute: 1996). Another staging system is the international TNM scale in which Tumor size (T), the extent of spread to the lymph Nodes (N), and the extent the cancer has spread or Metastasized (M) to other parts of the body are used to provide specific information about cancer stages (American Cancer Society: 1996).

In addition to staging, cancer cells are graded to determine how aggressive the tumor is. Grading measures how similar cancer cells are to normal cells. The more similar they are, the less aggressive the tumor. The Gleason system is the most common grading system. It ranges from a low score of 2 to a high score of 10. A Gleason score of 2 to 4 indicates that the cancer cells are less aggressive and usually slower to progress. An intermediate score is 5 to 7; a score of 8 to 10 predicts that the cancer cells are more likely to be aggressive (American Cancer Society: 1996).

Treatment Options

Treatment options vary depending on the individual's tumor stage, age, and his overall health. Prostate cancer is a very slow growing cancer; surgery is elective, not an emergency. Individuals whose tumors are confined to the prostate may choose to undergo a *radical prostatectomy*. This procedure is performed through a midline incision, from navel to pubic bone, or through the perineum. The entire prostate, the section of urethra that passes through it, and some of the surrounding tissue are removed from their position below the bladder. Pelvic lymph nodes may also be removed. The neck of the bladder is sutured to the remaining section of the urethra, and a catheter is inserted through the penis into the bladder to drain the urine while the wound heals. The catheter will remain in place for about 21 days following surgery. In the past, virtually all men who had this surgery became impotent. A nerve sparing technique is now used to preserve the nerves going to the penis so that potency may be maintained, although it may take 12 to 18 months for potency to return (Marks: 1995). The Prostate Cancer Outcomes Study looked at men diagnosed with primary prostate cancer between October, 1994 and October 1995 who underwent radical prostatectomy within six months of diagnosis. In the study, Stanford and colleagues (2000) found that 8.4% of the men were incontinent and nearly 60% were impotent at 18 months or more after the surgery. Of those men who were potent prior to surgery, the proportion who reported subsequent impotence varied due to the procedure used (56%, bilateral nerve-sparing; 58.6%, unilateral nerve-sparing; and 65.6%, non-nerve-sparing). In general, younger men who have had no erectile dysfunction prior to surgery do better post-surgically than older men who had experienced pre-surgical dysfunction. Laparoscopic prostatectomy, a new, minimally invasive procedure, is being used in a small number of U.S. medical centers. It is not yet known whether the procedure will significantly reduce the rates of incontinence or erectile dysfunction.

Incontinence is a common side effect of prostatectomy. The urinary sphincter muscle that controls urine outflow located below the prostate and the nerves that control it may be damaged when the prostate is removed. In overflow incontinence, the bladder retains urine after voiding and leaks involuntarily. Stress incontinence occurs when pressure to the bladder increases, usually during coughing, sneezing, exercise, and, sometimes, merely when rising from a chair or bed. Men with urge incontinence lose urine as soon as they feel the need to go to the bathroom. Some men find that incontinence is relieved with bladder training and pelvic muscle exercises. In bladder training, individuals learn to control the urge to urinate. They may also use a technique called prompted voiding or urinating on a schedule. Pelvic muscle exercises, also called Kegel exercises, strengthen pelvic muscles to hold back urine flow. During recuperation from surgery, incontinence products such as absorbent undergarments or pads may be used to manage incontinence. Men who continue to have severe incontinence may undergo urodynamic testing to evaluate bladder and sphincter function. The physician may suggest the use of a condom catheter or indwelling catheter, a penis clamp, or the surgical implantation of an artificial urinary sphincter.

The experiences of a writer who underwent surgery for prostate cancer provide an informative source for men who are contemplating surgery themselves. Korda (1996) was embarrassed to ask his doctor about a second opinion regarding treatment for prostate cancer; he worried that the physician would think that he did not trust him. When Korda consulted with a second urologist and showed him articles about patients' survival rates, the urologist became very angry. As in the case of Korda's physicians, urologists, radiation oncologists, and other specialists are likely to have biases for treatment based on their particular specialty; urologists recommend surgery, oncologists suggest radiation therapy. Different physicians gave Korda differing opinions as to the best course of treatment, yet he felt pressured to make a fast decision. Regardless of the treatment choice, these specialists agree that incontinence and erectile dysfunction are significant side effects (Barry: 2001).

Physicians often downplay the need for post-surgical care. Although Korda's physician told him that he would not need nursing care at home after prostate surgery, he found that he did need nursing care. His community home health agency gave him a list of practical supplies that he would require, such as waterproof pads, surgical dressings, and incontinence products, and provided a home health aide for personal care.

Another treatment option is *external radiation therapy*, in which a beam of radiation is aimed at the prostate in order to destroy cancer cells. Treatment is provided on an outpatient basis and usually extends six to eight weeks. External radiation may cause damage to rectal tissue. *Internal radiation therapy*, also called *interstitial brachytherapy*, is administered through radioactive seeds surgically implanted in the prostate, guided by transrectal ultrasound and computed tomography (CT) imaging. These seeds contain radioisotopes that emit rays for about three months. Rectal complications are rare, because the radiation is administered directly to the tumor. Many cancer centers use external radiation therapy rather than internal therapy to avoid the risks of surgery. The major side effects of either type of radiation therapy are fatigue, diarrhea, and painful urination, symptoms that appear during the latter part of treatment and improve over time. In addition, the nerves around the prostate and the arteries that carry blood to the penis are damaged by the radiation, leading to problems in achieving an erection. Forty to fifty percent of those treated with radiation therapy become impotent (National Cancer Institute: 1995). Men with symptoms of rectal bleeding and fecal discharge may have radiation proctitis, caused by damage to the tissue that lines the rectum. This condition is more likely in men with other health complications such as diabetes, high blood pressure, heart disease, or peripheral vascular disease (Bank: 1996). Laser treatment is used to reduce bleeding from rectal tissues, and a high fiber diet is recommended to improve stool formation.

When cancer has spread beyond the prostate to the lymph nodes or other parts of the body, *hormone therapy* is used to decrease the amount of testosterone, the male hormone that fuels the growth of the cancer cells. The testicles, a major source of testosterone, may be removed in a surgical procedure called an orchiectomy. The side effects of this surgery are impotence and hot flashes. A non-surgical alternative is an injection of drugs called luteinizing hormone releasing hormone analogs (LHRH) that shut down the production of testosterone. The injection can be given once a month or every three months. LHRH analogs can also cause hot flashes and impotence. An anti-androgen drug that blocks the action of testosterone in the adrenal gland may be used in conjunction with an LHRH analog. Its side effects include nausea, vomiting, diarrhea, hot flashes, and impotence. The female hormone, estrogen, is also used to suppress the supply of testosterone, although it can lead to cardiovascular problems such as blood clots and stroke. A study that analyzed the results of 24 randomized clinical trials concluded that survival rates were the same for men treated with surgery or LHRH (Seidenfeld et al.: 1999).

Chemotherapy is used to reduce pain and slow tumor growth in individuals with advanced prostate cancer, but it has not been found to be effective in achieving remission or stopping the spread of the disease (McDougal: 1996). Anti-cancer drugs are administered by injection or taken orally. Since these drugs flow throughout the body, the dosage and frequency must be monitored carefully to avoid damage to healthy cells. Chemotherapy treatments may be given in the hospital, physician's office, or at home. Many individuals experience side effects such as nausea, vomiting, anemia, hair loss, susceptibility to infection, and sores in the mouth.

The first national randomized controlled trial comparing watchful waiting with radical prostatectomy in men with prostate cancer will not report its results until 2008 (Agency for Health Care Policy and Research: 1997). Yet the results of a survey of urologists conducted by Plawker (1997) reveal that the majority of the survey respondents performed radical prostatectomies on men even if their age suggested that they would receive little benefit. Indicators such as PSA scores and Gleason staging were disregarded by the respondents. The findings of this study suggest that men should be especially wary when a surgeon recommends surgery for prostate cancer.

National health organizations such as the American Cancer Society and the National Cancer Institute provide information on cancer treatments, clinical trials, and community services. If possible, you should speak with others who have prostate cancer, possibly at support group meetings (see "ORGANIZATIONS" section below).

In order to make a wise decision about diagnosis and treatment for prostate cancer, men should consider the following:

• What does the current medical literature reveal about the accuracy of the PSA test as a predictor of prostate cancer? Have recent studies shown that the PSA test is useful in reducing deaths from prostate cancer? Have any more reliable diagnostic methods been developed?

• Do my PSA results and Gleason staging, considered in the context of my age and health condition, indicate that surgery would provide any benefit to me? Would other types of treatment be equally or more beneficial? Would my life span be increased by either surgical or medical treatment? If so, what would the quality of my life be like?

• Does the medical literature indicate that any new treatments have been developed that improve the survival rate for men with prostate cancer?

• Are there any preliminary data available from clinical trials currently underway that demonstrate a better cure rate with a specific treatment?

• Have other men that I have spoken to experienced post-surgical complications such as impotence and incontinence? If so, how long have these conditions lasted? Am I willing to take the risk of developing these complications? Have any new surgical techniques been developed that will improve the odds that I will not become impotent or incontinent?

• Have any drugs been approved that decrease the chances of impotence or incontinence? If so, what are their success rates and their side effects? What are the contraindications for taking these drugs (e.g., interactions with other drugs, dangerous for people who have certain illnesses)?

• Am I willing to accept incontinence or impotence and their effects on my quality of life in order to lengthen my life span? How would my partner feel about these choices?

• If I have prostate cancer and decide against treatment, how would it affect me psychologically? How would it affect my partner?

After considering these factors and others, men and the people closest to them should discuss the risks and benefits of the various options and make a decision based on the facts and the calculated risks. Decisions need not be final. Men who at one point opted for no treatment may later decide to have treatment if their condition progresses.

References

Agency for Health Care Policy and Research
1997 "Debate Continues Over Appropriate Treatment of BPH and Localized Prostate Cancer" Research Activities December Volume 211, pp. 6-8
American Cancer Society
1996 After Diagnosis: Prostate Cancer Atlanta, GA: American Cancer Society
1995a Facts on Prostate Cancer Atlanta, GA: American Cancer Society
1995b The PSA Blood Test and Prostate Cancer Atlanta, GA: American Cancer Society
American Medical Association
2000 "Screening and Early Detection of Prostate Cancer" Featured CSA (Council on Scientific Affairs Report www.ama-assn.org
Bank, Leslie
1996 "Radiation Proctitis--Cause and Treatment" Participate 5:2:3
Barry, Michael J.
2001 "Prostate-Specific-Antigen Testing for Early Diagnosis of Prostate Cancer" New England Journal of Medicine 344:18(May 3):1373-1377
Centers for Disease Control and Prevention
2001 Prostate Cancer: The Public Health Perspective 2001 Atlanta, GA: National Center for Chronic Disease Prevention and Health Promotion
Chabner, Bruce A. et al.
1997 "Screening Strategies for Cancer: Implications and Results" JAMA 277:18(May 14):1475
Collins, Mary McNaughton et al.
1997 "Medical Malpractice Implications of PSA Testing for Early Detection of Prostate Cancer" Journal of Law, Medicine & Ethics 25:4:234-242
Flood, A.B. et al.
1996 "The Importance of Patient Preference in the Decision to Screen for Prostate Cancer" Journal of General Internal Medicine 11(6):342-9
Korda, Michael
1996 Man to Man: Surviving Prostate Cancer Westminster, MD: Random House
Marks, Sheldon
1995 Prostate Cancer: A Family Guide to Diagnosis, Treatment and Survival Tucson, AZ: Fisher Books
McDougal, W. Scott
1996 Prostate Disease Westminster, MD: Random House
Mettlin, Curtis
1997 "The American Cancer Society National Prostate Cancer Detection Project and National Patterns of Prostate Cancer Detection and Treatment" CA: A Cancer Journal for Clinicians 47:5:265-273
National Cancer Institute
1996 PDQ State-of-The Art Cancer Treatment Summary for Patients: Prostate Cancer Washington, DC: National Cancer Institute

1995 <u>Prostate Cancer: Causes, Detection, Prevention, and Treatment</u> Washington, DC: National Cancer Institute

Plawker, Marc W.

1997 "Current Trends in Prostate Cancer Diagnosis and Staging among United States Urologists" <u>Journal of Urology</u> 158:1853-1858

Prostate Health Council

1998 <u>Important Information About Prostate-Specific Antigen (PSA)</u> Baltimore, MD: American Foundation for Urologic Disease, Inc.

1998 <u>Prostate Cancer: What Every Man 40 Should Know</u> Baltimore, MD: American Foundation for Urologic Disease, Inc.

Rose, Verna L.

1997 "ACP Issues Guidelines on the Early Detection of Prostate Cancer and Screening for Prostate Cancer" <u>American Family Physician</u> 56:6(October 15):1674

Seidenfeld, J. et al.

1999 "Single-Androgen Suppression in Men with Advanced Prostate Cancer: A Systematic Review and Meta-Analysis" <u>Annals of Internal Medicine</u> 132:7:566-577

Stanford, Janet L. et al.

2000 "Urinary and Sexual Function After Radical Prostatectomy for Clinically Localized Prostate Cancer" <u>JAMA</u> 283:3(January 19):354-360

ORGANIZATIONS

American Cancer Society (ACS)
1599 Clifton Road, NE
Atlanta, GA 30329
(800) 227-2345   www.cancer.org

This national voluntary health organization funds research and provides education, advocacy, and services to individuals with cancer, their families, and professionals. Produces many publications on prostate cancer including "For Men Only: What You Should Know About Prostate Cancer," "The PSA Blood Test and Prostate Cancer," and "Facts On Prostate Cancer." Free

American Foundation for Urologic Disease (AFUD)
1128 North Charles Street
Baltimore, MD 21201
(800) 242-2383   (410) 468-1800   FAX (410) 468-1808
e-mail: admin@afud.org   www.afud.org

Supports research, education, and patient support services, including the Prostate Cancer Support Network. Sponsors annual low cost or free prostate cancer screenings. Membership, $35.00, includes subscription to quarterly magazine, "FAMILY Urology," and quarterly newsletter, "Foundation Focus."

American Prostate Society
7188 Ridge Road
Hanover, MD 21076
(410) 859-3735   FAX (410) 850-0818
e-mail: webmaster@www.ameripros.org
www.ameripros.org

Provides education about prostate diseases and treatment. Quarterly newsletter, "Update," free. Membership is free.

Cancer Care, Inc.
275 Seventh Avenue
New York, NY 10001
National Toll-free Counseling Line (800) 813-4673
(212) 302-2400   e-mail: info@cancercare.org
www.cancercare.org

The national toll-free counseling line offers psychological support to individuals with cancer and their families. Social workers also provide information and referral to community resources, educational materials, guidelines for doctor-patient communication, and telephone support groups. Direct services, such as financial assistance to help with costs of home care and transportation, are provided nationwide. The "Helping Hand Resource Guide" is an online database of national and regional organizations. All services are free.

Cancer Information Center, National Cancer Institute (NCI)
31 Center Drive, MSC 2580
Building 31, Room 10A03
Bethesda, MD 20892-2580
(800) 422-6237   FAX (301) 330-7968   www.nci.nih.gov

Provides information on many types of cancer, treatment, resource organizations, and publications, including "Publications for Cancer Patients and the Public." Free. Also publishes self-help guides such as "Radiation Therapy and You," "Chemotherapy and You," "Pain Control: A Guide for People with Cancer and Their Families," and "Facing Forward: A Guide for Cancer Survivors." All publications are free. Spanish-speaking staff members available. Calling the "800" phone number listed above connects with the regional center closest to you, which can provide information about the resources described above as well as local resources.

Impotence World Institute (IWA)
119 South Ruth Street
Maryville, TN 37803
(800) 669-1603   (865) 379-2154
e-mail: info@impotenceworld.org   www.impotenceworld.org

A membership organization with support groups throughout the country. Operates a help line and makes referrals to physicians. Membership, $25.00, includes quarterly newsletter, "Impotence Worldwide."

Man to Man: Prostate Cancer Education and Support Program
American Cancer Society (ACS)
1599 Clifton Road, NE
Atlanta, GA 30329
(800) 227-2345   www.cancer.org

This program provides practical information and emotional support to men who have been diagnosed with prostate cancer and their families. Produces quarterly "Man to Man Newsletter;" free. Call toll-free number to request information about this program in local areas.

MEDLINEplus: Prostate Cancer
www.nlm.nih.gov/medlineplus/prostatecancer

This web site provides links to sites for general information about prostate cancer, prevention and screening, symptoms and diagnosis, treatment, alternative therapy, clinical trials, statistics, organizations, journals and newsletters, and coping with prostate cancer. An interactive tutorial on radiation therapy for prostate cancer is available at www.nlm.nih.gov/medlineplus/tutorials

National Association for Continence (NAFC)
PO Box 8310
Spartanburg, SC 29305-8310
(800) 252-3337   (864) 579-7900   FAX (864) 579-7902
www.nafc.org

An information clearinghouse for consumers, family members, and medical professionals. Will answer individual questions if self-addressed stamped envelope is enclosed with letter. Membership, $20.00, includes a quarterly newsletter, "Quality Care," a "Resource Guide: Products and Services for Continence" (nonmembers, $13.00), discount on publications, and a continence resource service. Free publications list.

National Cancer Data Base
American College of Surgeons
www.facs.org

Reports on oncology outcomes at 1600 hospitals in 50 states. Annotated bibliographies and cancer statistics may be downloaded from web site.

National Cancer Institute (NCI)
Physician Data Query (PDQ)
CancerNet
CANCERLIT
LiveHelp
31 Center Drive MSC 2580
Building 31, Room 10A03
Bethesda, MD 20892
(800) 422-6237   (800) 332-8615 (TT)   FAX (301) 402-5874
CancerFax (800) 624-2511   e-mail: cancermail@cips.nci.nih.gov
cancer.gov

The National Cancer Institute supports basic and clinical research investigations into the causes, prevention, and cure for cancer. The PDQ database provides up-to-date information on cancer prevention, screening, treatments, and care. PDQ is available on the Internet through CancerNet, which also contains fact sheets and publications, CancerNet news, and CANCERLIT abstracts and citations. CancerFax provides access by fax machine to information statements from the PDQ Database, CANCERLIT citations and abstracts, and fact sheets on cancer topics. LiveHelp is a pilot program that provides live, online assistance from an NCI Information Specialist; available Monday-Friday, 12-4 pm, Eastern Time. Most information is also available in Spanish. Calling the "800" phone number listed above connects with the regional center closest to you, which can provide information about the resources described above as well as local resources.

National Kidney and Urologic Diseases Information Clearinghouse (NKUDIC)
3 Information Way
Bethesda, MD 20892
(800) 891-5390   (301) 654-4415
e-mail: nkudic@info.niddk.nih.gov
www.niddk.nih.gov/health/kidney/nkudic.htm

Responds to requests from the public and professionals about impotence and prostate conditions. Maintains a publications database. Free list of publications.

National Prostate Cancer Coalition (NPCC)
1158 15th Street, NW
Washington, DC 20005
(888) 245-9455   (202) 463-9455   FAX (202) 463-9456
e-mail: info@4npcc.org   www.4npcc.org

This advocacy organization lobbies for funding for prostate cancer research. A newsletter, "Smart Brief," is published by e-mail each Tuesday and Friday.

PACCT-PCOG (Patient Advocates for Advanced Cancer Treatments-Prostate Cancer Oncology Group)
1143 Parmelee, NW
Grand Rapids, MI 49504
(616) 453-1477   FAX (616) 453-1846
e-mail: paact@naxnet-usa.net   www.paactusa.org

This patient advocacy organization provides information about detection, diagnosis, and treatment options. Membership, $50.00, includes quarterly newsletter, "Cancer Communication." Newsletter also available on the web site.

Prostate.com
TAP Pharmaceutical, Inc.
675 North Field Drive
Lake Forest, IL 60045
(800) 621-1020   www.tap.com   www.prostate.com

This web site, sponsored by a manufacturer of hormonal therapy for prostate cancer, offers basic information about prostate diseases, treatments, and living with prostate cancer. Site offers "What To Ask Your Doctor About Prostate Cancer," a form that may be printed and taken to medical appointments.

Simon Foundation for Continence
PO Box 835
Wilmette, IL 60091
(800) 237-4666   (847) 864-3913   FAX (847) 864-9758
e-mail: simoninfo@simonfoundation.org
www.simonfoundation.org

Provides information and assistance to people who are incontinent. Organizes self-help groups. Membership, individuals, $15.00; professionals, $35.00; includes quarterly newsletter, "The Informer." Also available on the web site.

US TOO! International, Inc.
5003 Fairview Avenue
Downers Grove, IL 60515
(800) 808-7866   (630) 795-1002   FAX (630) 795-1602
e-mail: ustoo@ustoo.com   www.ustoo.com

This international support network of chapters links prostate cancer survivors, families, and health care professionals. Sponsors US TOO! Partners support groups. Membership, $25.00, includes quarterly newsletter, "The US TOO Prostate Cancer Communicator." A daily e-mail newsletter, "Prostate Cancer News You Can Use" is available. Free

YourSurgery.com
yoursurgery.com

This multimedia site uses simple diagrams and animation to show how a prostatectomy is performed. Click on "Pelvis," then on "prostatectomy."

About Prostatectomy
American College of Surgeons
633 North Saint Clare Street
Chicago, IL 60611
(312) 202-5000   FAX (312) 202-5001
e-mail: postmaster@facs.org   www.facs.org

This brochure describes this surgical procedure. Free. Also available on the web site.

After Diagnosis: Prostate Cancer
American Cancer Society (ACS)
1599 Clifton Road, NE
Atlanta, GA 30329
(800) 227-2345   www.cancer.org

This booklet discusses the diagnosis of prostate cancer, staging and grading of tumors, and treatment options such as surgery, radiation, and hormone therapy and their side effects. Includes glossary and resource guide. Free

Before, During, and After Your Radical Prostatectomy
American Foundation for Urologic Disease (AFUD)
1128 North Charles Street
Baltimore, MD 21201
(800) 242-2383   (410) 468-1800   FAX (410) 468-1808
e-mail: admin@afud.org   www.afud.org

This booklet discusses pre-operative tests, surgical details, pain control, and post-operative care. Free

Everyone's Guide to Cancer Therapy
by Malin Dollinger, Ernest H. Rosenbaum, and Greg Cable
Andrews and McMeel
PO Box 419150
Kansas City, MO 64141
(800) 642-6480

This book describes the diagnosis, treatment, and daily management of common cancers, including prostate cancer. Includes chapters on treatment options, supportive care, sexuality, improving quality of life, and new advances in research, diagnosis, and treatment. Provides a glossary of medical terms, and lists of anticancer drugs and their side effects, cancer associations and support groups, comprehensive cancer care centers, clinical trials sites, and suggested reading. $21.95 plus $4.25 shipping and handling

Harvard Men's Health Watch
PO Box 420099
Palm Coast, FL 32142
(800) 829-5921   e-mail: harvardmed@palmcoastd.com
www.health.harvard.edu/newsletters

This monthly newsletter reports on men's health issues, including prostate conditions, screening, diagnosis, and treatments. $24.00

Important Information About Prostate-Specific Antigen (PSA)
Prostate Health Council
American Foundation for Urologic Disease (AFUD)
1128 North Charles Street
Baltimore, MD 21201
(800) 242-2383   (410) 468-1800   FAX (410) 468-1808
e-mail: admin@afud.org   www.afud.org

This booklet discusses testing for the prostate-specific antigen (PSA) found in blood. Free

A Man's Guide to Coping with Disability
Resources for Rehabilitation
33 Bedford Street, Suite 19A
Lexington, MA 02420
(781) 862-6455   FAX (781) 861-7517   e-mail: info@rfr.org
www.rfr.org

This book includes information about men's responses to disability, with a special emphasis on the values men place on independence, occupational achievement, and physical activity. Information on finding local services, self-help groups, laws that affect men with disabilities, sports and recreation, and employment is applicable to men with any type of disability or chronic condition. Chapters on prostate conditions, coronary heart disease, diabetes, HIV/AIDS, multiple sclerosis, spinal cord injury, and stroke include information about the disease or condition, psychological aspects, sexual functioning, where to find services, environmental adaptations, and annotated entries of organizations, publications and tapes, and resources for assistive devices. Includes e-mail addresses and Internet resources. $44.95 plus $5.00 shipping and handling (See last page of this book for order form.)

Man to Man: Surviving Prostate Cancer
by Michael Korda
Random House
400 Hahn Road, PO Box 100
Westminster, MD 21157
(800) 733-3000   (410) 848-1900   FAX (410) 386-7013
www.randomhouse.com

Written by a prostate cancer survivor, this book describes the author's experiences receiving his diagnosis and choosing surgical treatment, undergoing radical prostatectomy, and coping with side effects such as incontinence and impotence. $13.00 plus $5.50 shipping and handling

Men, Women and Prostate Cancer: A Medical and Psychological Guide for Women and the Men They Love
by Barbara Rubin Wainrib and Sandra Haber with Jack Maguire
New Harbinger Publications, Inc.
5674 Shattuck Avenue
Oakland, CA 94609
(800) 748-6273   (510) 652-0215   FAX (510) 652-5472
www.newharbinger.com

This book discusses the detection and diagnosis of prostate cancer and offers suggestions for dealing with both practical and emotional aspects of the diagnosis. It describes treatment options and strategies for coping with treatment, impotence, incontinence, and sexual concerns. $15.95

The Prostate: A Guide for Men and the Women Who Love Them
by Patrick C. Walsh and Janet Farrar Worthington
Johns Hopkins University Press
PO Box 50370
Baltimore, MD 21211-4370
(800) 537-5487   FAX (410) 516-6998   www.press.jhu.edu/press

Written by a urologist and a science writer, this book discusses prostate cancer, benign prostatic hyperplasia, and prostatitis. Describes diagnosis, treatments, and side effects, such as impotence. Includes a glossary. $15.95 plus $4.00 shipping and handling

The Prostate Book
by Stephen N. Rous
W. W. Norton & Company
800 Keystone Industrial Park
Scranton, PA 18512
(800) 223-2588   (717) 346-2029   FAX (800) 458-6515
www.wwnorton.com

Written by a urologist, this book describes the anatomy and function of the prostate as well as diagnosis and treatment of prostatitis, BPH, and prostate cancer. Complications and side effects of treatment are also discussed. Includes a glossary. Hardcover, $26.95; softcover, $13.00.

Prostate Cancer: A Non-Surgical Perspective
by Kent Wallner
Pathways Book Service
4 White Brook Road
Gilsum, NH 03448
(800) 345-6665   e-mail: pbs@pathwaybook.com

This book, written by a radiation oncologist, describes and compares treatment options, listing side effects and complications. Includes chapter on impotence. Large print. $18.95

Prostate Cancer Resource Guide
American Foundation for Urologic Disease (AFUD)
1128 North Charles Street
Baltimore, MD 21201
(800) 242-2383   (410) 468-1800   FAX (410) 468-1808
e-mail: admin@afud.org   www.afud.org

This booklet discusses treatment choices and lists prostate cancer support groups, resource organizations, and publications. Includes prostate cancer bibliography. $5.00

Prostate Cancer: The Public Health Perspective 2001
Centers for Disease Control and Prevention (CDC)
National Center for Chronic Disease Prevention and Health Promotion
Mail Stop K-64
4770 Buford Highway, NE
Atlanta, GA 30341
(888) 842-6355   (770) 488-4751   FAX (770) 488-4760
e-mail: cancerinfo@cdc.gov   www.cdc.gov/cancer

This publication provides an overview of the controversy over early detection and treatment and describes the CDC's activities that target prostate cancer. Free. Also available on the web site.

Prostate Cancer Treatment Guidelines for Patients
National Comprehensive Cancer Network (NCCN)
50 Huntingdon Pike, Suite 200
Rockledge, PA 19046
(888) 909-6226   (215) 728-4788   FAX (215) 728-3877
e-mail: patientinformation@nccn.org
www.nccn.org/patient/guidelines

These guidelines, developed by the NCCN and the American Cancer Society, are based on NCCN Oncology Practice Guidelines. Available in English and Spanish. Also available on the NCCN web site and the American Cancer Society web site: www.cancer.org

Prostate Cancer: What Every Man Over 40 Should Know
Prostate Health Council
American Foundation for Urologic Disease (AFUD)
1128 North Charles Street
Baltimore, MD 21201
(800) 242-2383   (410) 468-1800   FAX (410) 468-1808
e-mail: admin@afud.org   www.afud.org

This booklet provides information about symptoms and diagnosis of prostate cancer. Available in English and Spanish. Free. Also available on the web site.

Sexuality and Cancer: For the Man Who Has Cancer and His Partner
by Leslie Schover
American Cancer Society (ACS)
1599 Clifton Road, NE
Atlanta, GA 30329
(800) 227-2345   www.cancer.org

This booklet discusses the effects of cancer treatment on male sexuality, suggests strategies for dealing with sexual problems, and describes sources for professional help and additional publications. American Cancer Society service programs are listed, including self-help support groups. Free

Sexuality and Fertility After Cancer
by Leslie Schover
John Wiley and Sons
1 Wiley Drive
Somerset, NJ 08875
(800) 225-5945   (732) 469-4400   www.wiley.com

This book answers common questions about sexuality and fertility asked by cancer survivors, their partners, and families. Topics include men's sexual health, erectile dysfunction, and prostate cancer. Includes resource list. $15.95 plus $5.00 shipping and handling

Teamwork: The Cancer Patient's Guide to Talking with Your Doctor
by Elizabeth J. Clark (ed.)
National Coalition for Cancer Survivorship (NCCS)
1010 Wayne Avenue, Suite 770
Silver Spring, MD 20910
(877) 622-7937   (301) 650-9127   FAX (301) 565-9670
e-mail: info@cansearch.org   www.cansearch.org

This publication provides practical suggestions to help people with cancer communicate with their doctors. Based on the experience of individuals with cancer, it includes questions that they should ask and information the doctor should get from them. Available in English and Spanish. Free plus $2.00 shipping and handling

Treatment Choices for Localized Prostate Cancer
American Foundation for Urologic Disease (AFUD)
1128 North Charles Street
Baltimore, MD 21201
(800) 242-2383   (410) 468-1800   FAX (410) 468-1808
e-mail: admin@afud.org   www.afud.org

This booklet discusses the staging and treatment of prostate cancer. It describes tests such as biopsy and computed tomography (CT) scans and surgical, radiologic, and hormonal treatments. Free

Two Against One: A Spouse's Guide to Coping with Prostate Cancer
US TOO! International, Inc.
(877) 550-9624   www.2against1.com

This booklet provides basic information about prostate cancer, describes the emotions that accompany a cancer diagnosis, and suggests strategies for coping. Includes a resource list. Free

Urinary Incontinence
National Institute on Aging Information Center
PO Box 8057
Gaithersburg, MD 20898-8057
(800) 222-2225   e-mail: niaic@jbs1.com   www.nih.gov/nia/health

This brochure discusses the types, treatment, and management of urinary incontinence. Large print. Free. Also available on the web site.

What You Need to Know about Prostate Cancer
Cancer Information Center, National Cancer Institute (NCI)
31 Center Drive MSC 2580
Building 31, Room 10A03
Bethesda, MD 20892
(800) 422-6237   (800) 332-8615 (TT)   FAX (301) 402-5874
CancerFax (800) 624-2511   e-mail: cancermail@cips.nci.nih.gov
cancer.gov

This booklet, written for patients and their families, discusses symptoms, diagnosis, staging, treatment methods and side effects, and follow-up care associated with prostate cancer. A list of medical terms and resources is also included. Free

Wrongful Death
by Sandra M. Gilbert
W. W. Norton & Company
Keystone Industrial Park
Scranton, PA 18512
(800) 223-2588   (717) 346-2029   FAX (800) 458-6515
www.wwnorton.com

Written by a woman whose husband died after routine prostate surgery, this book examines her shock and grief and the decision to sue the hospital for medical negligence. Hardcover, $22.50; softcover, $13.00; plus $4.00 shipping and handling.

Your Choice for Treating Prostate Cancer
TAP Pharmaceuticals, Inc.
675 North Field Drive
Lake Forest, IL 60045
(800) 621-1020   www.tap.com   www.prostate.com

This videotape describes palliative hormone treatment for advanced prostate cancer. Single copy, free.

Chapter 11

TERMINAL ILLNESS

When individuals receive the diagnosis of a terminal illness, quite understandably, both they and their families are in a state of shock. At the very time that they are in need of the greatest amount of emotional support, they are least likely to get it from the medical community. When physicians are unable to cure a disease, they feel powerless and purposely distance themselves from their patients (Mizrahi: 1986).

Physicians dealing with terminally ill patients should give full information about the prognosis to the patient and his or her family, so that they may make informed decisions about treatments. While some individuals may opt for aggressive treatment, even when the probability that they will recover is minimal, others will opt for palliative care, to maintain a maximum level of comfort without any attempt to prolong life. In either case, physicians should respect the patient's decision, be understanding of the emotions of both the patient and family members, and provide comfort and adequate pain control. Emanuel and colleagues (2000) interviewed the caregivers of nearly 1000 terminally ill individuals about the emotional and physical stresses of caregiving. Those whose physicians listened to their concerns and feelings about their loved one and the challenges of caregiving felt less stress.

Decisions about the type of care that should be provided in the final stage of life should be reached jointly by the individual and his or her family and significant others based on information about the condition and its effects, along with possible treatment options. The physician should provide information about the condition, along with references to literature, voluntary organizations, and support systems. The advantages of advance directives and health care proxies become apparent if the individual is no longer mentally capable of making decisions.

The decision about aggressive treatment versus palliative care is a very personal choice. Some individuals desire aggressive treatment, vowing never to give up no matter what the odds. Others in similar situations tranquilly accept the fact that they are dying and prefer maximum pain control over aggressive treatment. They may leave orders for the medical staff not to resuscitate them. It is a person's right to refuse treatment at any point. A physician may not insist upon aggressive treatment if the patient refuses. The patient and his or her advocate should always question the benefits of any procedure and the quality of life that will ensue.

If a physician recommends immediate surgery or other procedures, you should question whether delaying the procedure will result in a likely difference in the outcome. In most cases, it will not. In advanced cases of cancer, for example, surgery may prolong life by weeks or months or result in relief of pain, but it will not cure the disease. Having a week or so to research the condition and the various treatment options will allow for a rational decision and the reassurance that you chose the right option. The extra time also enables you to get second and possibly third opinions. A physician who pressures you into making an immediate decision may have ulterior motives (i.e., making sure that you do not have surgery performed by another surgeon), unless the situation is truly an emergency. In a time of great emotional stress, individuals and advocates must use all their ability to remain calm and use their energy to get all of the necessary information to make a wise decision.

A study of residents of long term care facilities (Wetle et al.: 1988) found that most of the respondents (61.4%) would want to be involved in "do not resuscitate" decisions. Despite their wishes to be involved in this decision, nearly all of the respondents (92.6%) claimed that they had never been asked about resuscitation. In order to avoid this situation and remain involved in decisions regarding your own care, use an advance directive to make your wishes known regarding pain control, palliative care, resuscitation, and many other health care decisions (see Chapter 5, "ADVANCE DIRECTIVES" section).

HOSPICE PROGRAMS

In the past two decades, hospice programs have gained widespread acceptance in the United States. Hospice care is based on the notion that individuals with terminal illnesses should be allowed to have a death with dignity and with maximum pain control. Quality of life takes precedence over length of life, with no extraordinary measures taken to extend a patient's life. However, measures are taken to help the person enjoy his or her remaining days, and palliative care to maximize physical comfort is provided by medical personnel. Hospice care is available to children as well as adults.

Hospice programs take a variety of forms, from inpatient residential care to home care. Hospice programs are sometimes independent programs, sometimes operated under the auspices of a hospital or nursing home facility, and sometimes part of an organization such as a visiting nurses agency. Services are available 24 hours a day, 7 days a week. Hospice programs include not only health care personnel, but counselors and members of the clergy. Family members and other close friends of the dying person may benefit from grief counseling provided by hospice for up to a year after the person's death.

Medicare now pays for hospice services, if a physician certifies that the individual has a life-threatening illness and has six months or less to live. The individual must sign a statement indicating that he or she chooses hospice care rather than standard medical care for the illness. The Medicare Hospice Benefit provides four levels of care: routine home care, continuous home care, inpatient respite care and general inpatient care. Services covered include those of a physician; nurse; occupational, physical, and speech-language therapists; drugs; counseling; respite care; and medical supplies and appliances. Medicare hospice care will pay only for pain control and symptom management; patients are responsible for a maximum of $5.00 per prescription. Inpatient respite care of up to five days is available in order to provide relief for the patient's caregiver; the patient is charged about $5.00 a day for this care. Special hospice benefit periods apply, including two 90 day periods, followed by an indefinite number of 60 day benefit periods. To determine the location of hospice care programs approved by Medicare, call the Medicare Hotline at (800) 633-4227. In some states, Medicaid will pay for hospice care. Most private insurance carriers and HMOs also cover hospice services. An individual may leave a hospice program voluntarily at any time; Medicare benefits are automatically restored without a waiting period.

Despite the finding that nearly two-thirds of patients prefer care that will keep them comfortable rather than prolong life, hospice programs are used in only ten percent of all cases of terminal illness (Lynn et al.: 1997). Health care professionals often delay making referrals for hospice care due to their own discomfort in moving from curing to caring for the patient; discussing end-of-life issues; concerns about a family's ability to provide home care; and lack of knowledge of hospice services. One-fifth of hospice patients die within a week of referral, and fifty percent within a month (American Hospice Foundation: 1998). Although physical comfort may be achieved through pain management in this interval, there is little time to deal with emotional and spiritual needs.

PAIN CONTROL DURING TERMINAL ILLNESS
(Also see Chapter 6, "Drugs")

Appropriate pain control during terminal illness has been the topic of much discussion over the past decades. Despite the knowledge that has been developed to help patients with intractable pain regain substantial levels of comfort, many, if not most, patients with diseases like cancer spend their final days, weeks, or even months in excruciating pain that could have been controlled. Physicians often do not believe their patients' descriptions of their pain, fail to assess patients' pain, and do not have a good understanding of pain control techniques (Cherny and Portenoy: 1994).

A study (Lynn et al.: 1997) found that most patients preferred treatment to keep them comfortable, even if it meant a shorter life; despite this preference, over half of all patients received aggressive treatment to prolong their lives, including feeding tubes, artificial respirators, or an attempt at cardiopulmonary resuscitation. Family members reported that 40% of the patients had severe pain most or all of the time in their last three days of life.

Knowledgeable medical consumers and their advocates should be able to overcome the problem of physicians who are unwilling to administer appropriate pain control because of the unrealistic fear that the patient will become a drug addict. Physicians also fear disciplinary action against them if they use high doses of narcotics, but they do not fear any legal action against them if they undertreat patients' pain (Tucker: 1998). By learning about the current protocols for pain control administration and discussing them with the physician, medical consumers and their advocates should be able to reach a joint decision about pain control. In the event that the physician is still reluctant to administer proper pain control, contact a hospice physician or a pain control center in order to obtain satisfaction. Some anesthesiology departments in hospitals operate pain control programs.

VIATICAL SETTLEMENTS

A viatical settlement is a little known financial option for individuals who are terminally ill. In order to finance medical procedures and care that may improve their quality of life, individuals who are terminally ill may decide to sell their life insurance policies for a cash settlement to a viatical settlement company. In return, the viatical settlement company receives the proceeds of the policy when the individual dies. In general, the insurance policy may be individually owned or part of a group policy, must have been in force for at least two years, and must not be subject to contestability. The Kennedy-Kassebaum Health Insurance Portability and Accountability Act exempts most viatical settlements from federal income tax. If you are considering a viatical settlement, you should check to determine tax liability, such as capital gains tax, on the proceeds of such a settlement and whether or not the settlement amount will affect income eligibility for state or federal entitlement programs. About a third of the states require that viatical settlement companies be licensed or registered. It is wise to consult an attorney when considering a viatical settlement and to compare at least three offers from different viatical companies.

Other methods of receiving benefits from a life insurance policy while the insured is living include borrowing against the cash value of the policy, cashing out the policy, or borrowing money, using the policy as collateral. Some life insurance companies offer "accelerated benefits" riders that pay policy benefits before the policyholder's death. Policyholders may pay an additional premium when the rider is added, or they pay when the option is used. Benefits are usually reduced to offset the insurance company's loss of interest when an early payout is made.

References

American Hospice Foundation
1998 Talking About Hospice Washington, DC: American Hospice Foundation
Cherny, N.I. and R.K. Portenoy
1994 "The Management of Cancer Pain" CA: A Cancer Journal for Clinicians
        44:5(September/October):263-303
Emanuel, Ezekiel J. et al.
2000 "Understanding Economic and Other Burdens of Terminal Illness: The Experience of
        Patients and Their Caregivers" Annals of Internal Medicine 132:6(March 21):451-459
Lynn, Joanne et al.
1997 "Perceptions by Family Members of the Dying Experience of Older and Seriously Ill
        Patients" Annals of Internal Medicine 126:2(January 15):97-105
Mizrahi, Terry
1986 Getting Rid of Patients New Brunswick, NJ: Rutgers University Press
Tucker, Kathryn L.
1998 "Treatment of Pain in Dying Patients" New England Journal of Medicine 338:17(April
        23):1231
Wetle, Terrie et al.
1988 "Nursing Home Resident Participation in Medical Decisions: Perceptions and
        Preferences" The Gerontologist 28(Suppl.):32-38

ORGANIZATIONS

American Academy of Hospice and Palliative Medicine (AAHPM)
4700 West Lake Avenue
Glenview, IL 60025
(847) 375-4712   FAX (877) 734-8671
e-mail: aahpm@aahpm.org   www.aahpm.org

An organization of physicians that works to promote hospice and palliative care through publications and symposia. Membership, $225.00, includes newsletter, "AAHPM Bulletin."

American Cancer Society (ACS)
1599 Clifton Road, NE
Atlanta, GA 30329
(800) 227-2345   www.cancer.org

This national voluntary health organization funds research and provides education, advocacy, and services to individuals with cancer, their families, and professionals. Produces many self-help guides, such as "Pain Control: A Guide for People with Cancer" and "Facing Forward: A Guide for Cancer Survivors." Many publications are free.

American Foundation for AIDS Research (AmFAR)
120 Wall Street, 13th floor
New York, NY 10005
(800) 392-6327   (212) 806-1600   FAX (212) 806-1601
e-mail: amfar@amfar.org   www.amfar.org

Funds basic biomedical research; operates the Community-Based Clinical Trials Network which enables physicians across the country to enroll patients in trials of new drugs and new therapies; and funds education for AIDS prevention. Publishes "The AMFAR Report" and "The AmFAR Newsletter."

American Heart Association (AHA)
7272 Greenville Avenue
Dallas, TX 75231
(800) 242-8721   (214) 373-6300   FAX (214) 706-1341
www.amhrt.org

Promotes research and education and publishes professional and public education brochures. Local affiliates. Membership fees vary.

American Hospice Foundation (AHF)
2120 L Street, NW, Suite 200
Washington, DC 20037
(202) 223-0204   FAX (202) 223-0208
e-mail: ahf@msn.com   www.americanhospice.org

An organization dedicated to improving access to hospice services by conducting outreach programs to increase public awareness of hospice.

Americans for Better Care of the Dying (ABCD)
4125 Albermarle Street, NW, Suite 210
Washington, DC 20016
(202) 895-9485   FAX (202) 895-9484
e-mail: info@abcd-caring.org   www.abcd-caring.com

This organization advocates for reform in end of life care. Membership, $50.00, includes newsletter, "ABCD Exchange," and a copy of "Promises to Keep: Changing the Way We Provide Care at the End of Life." Online resource list includes topics such as caregiving, end of life issues, hospice, palliative care, grief and bereavement, and pain management.

Cancer Care, Inc.
275 Seventh Avenue
New York, NY 10001
National Toll-free Counseling Line (800) 813-4673
(212) 302-2400   FAX (212) 719-0263
e-mail: info@cancercare.org   www.cancercare.org

The national toll-free counseling line offers psychological support to individuals with cancer and their families. Social workers also provide information and referral to community resources, educational materials, guidelines for doctor-patient communication, and telephone support groups. Direct services, such as financial assistance to help with costs of home care and transportation, are provided nationwide. The "Helping Hand Resource Guide" is an online database of national and regional organizations. All services are free.

Cancer Information Center, National Cancer Institute (NCI)
31 Center Drive, MSC 2580
Building 31, Room 10A03
Bethesda, MD 20892
(800) 422-6237   FAX (301) 330-7968   www.nci.nih.gov

Provides information on many types of cancer, treatment, resource organizations, and publications, including "Publications for Cancer Patients and the Public." Free. Spanish-speaking staff members available. Calling the "800" phone number listed above connects with the regional center closest to you, which can provide information about the resources described above as well as local resources.

CDC National Prevention Information Network (CDC NPIN)
PO Box 6003
Rockville, MD 20849
(800) 458-5231   (800) 243-7012 (TT)   FAX (888) 282-7681
e-mail: info@cdcnpin.org   www.cdcnpin.org

NPIN provides HIV and AIDS information, referrals, and publications. Spanish and French information specialists are also available.

CDC National STD and AIDS Hotline
(800) 342-2437   (800) 344-7432 (Spanish)
(800) 243-7889 (TT)

This 24 hour hot-line provides information about HIV transmission and prevention, HIV testing and treatment, referrals, and educational materials. Special resources are available for minorities and women. Spanish information specialists are bilingual and bicultural. Publications available in English and Spanish. Free

Children's Hospice International (CHI)
2202 Mt. Vernon Avenue, Suite 3C
Alexandria, VA 22301
(800) 242-4453   (703) 684-0330   FAX (703) 684-0226
e-mail: chiorg@aol.com   www.chionline.org

Promotes hospice support for children with life-threatening illnesses. Membership, individuals, $45.00; professionals, $65.00; includes quarterly newsletter and discounts on publications and conference registration. Free publications list.

Children's Oncology Group (COG)
440 East Huntington Drive, Suite 300
Arcadia, CA 91006
(626) 447-0064   FAX (626) 445-4334   www.nccf.org/cog

This collaborative national pediatric research group conducts clinical trials of new therapies for childhood cancer.

City of Hope Pain/Palliative Care Resource Center
1500 East Duarte Road
Duarte, CA 91010
(626) 359-8111, extension 63829   FAX (626) 301-8941
e-mail: mayday-pain@coh.org   mayday.coh.org

This national clearinghouse provides information on pain management for individuals and professionals. A Resource List that include organizations, videotapes, audiocassettes, and print publications is available free plus $3.00 shipping and handling. Also available on the web site.

Growth House, Inc.
(415) 255-9045   e-mail: info@growthhouse.org
www.growthhouse.org

Provides information and referral services for agencies working on death and dying issues. Directs users to resources for care for the dying; offers comprehensive guides for AIDS and cancer; and sites for resources on bereavement and grief.

Hospice Association of America
228 7th Street, SE
Washington, DC 20003
(202) 546-4759   www.hospice-america.org

Trade association which represents hospices, caregivers, and volunteers. It is an affiliate of the National Association of Home Care (NAHC). Offers general information to consumers. Also available on the web site.

Hospice Foundation of America (HFA)
2001 S Street NW, Suite 300
Washington, DC 20009
(800) 854-3402   (202) 638-5419   FAX (202) 638-5312
e-mail: hfa@hospicefoundation.org www.hospicefoundation.org

Promotes the hospice concept of care and conducts public education and professional education programs. Provides information about hospice care, how to select a hospice and how to locate a nearby hospice. Holds an annual bereavement teleconference. Publishes a newsletter, "Journeys," that provides advice on dealing with grief. $12.00.

Hospice Hands Links
hospicecares.com

Provides information for individuals and families considering hospice care as well as links to sites for pain management, children, and resource organizations.

HOSPICELINK
Hospice Education Institute
190 Westbrook Road
Essex, CT 06426
(800) 331-1620   (860) 767-1620   FAX (860) 767-2746
e-mail: hospiceAll@aol.com   www.hospiceworld.org

Promotes hospice care through publications and seminars and provides free information and referrals to hospice and palliative care programs.

Hospice Web
www.teleport.com/~hospice/links.htm

Provides a list of links and information about hospice providers by state and country.

Last Acts
1951 Kidwell Drive, Suite 205
Vienna, VA 22182
(703) 827-8771   www.lastacts.org

This coalition of organizations works to raise awareness of issues regarding death and dying. Offers families an online resource directory and electronic newsletter. Offers professionals an online journal, "Innovations in End-Of-Life Care," an online newsletter, and information about programs across the country.

Mended Hearts
7272 Greenville Avenue
Dallas, TX 75231
(800) 242-8721   (214) 706-1442   FAX (214) 706-5231
e-mail: mhoffice@heart.org   www.mendedhearts.org

This affiliate of the American Heart Association has chapters in many states. It offers support to individuals with heart disease through monthly meetings, raises funds for medical equipment and scholarships, offers an Internet Visiting Program, and trains volunteers to visit individuals who have undergone heart surgery. Membership, individuals, $17.00; families, $24.00; includes quarterly newsletter, "HEARTBEAT."

National Association for Home Care (NAHC)
228 7th Street, SE
Washington, DC 20003
(202) 547-7424   FAX (202) 547-3540   www.nahc.org

Trade association of home care and hospice organizations. Consumer education publications include "Information About Hospice: A Consumer's Guide" and the "Hospice Bill of Rights." Single copy, free. Also available on the web site.

National Association for People with AIDS (NAPWA)
1413 K Street, NW, 7th floor
Washington, DC 20006
(202) 898-0414   FAX (202) 898-0435
www.napwa.org

Promotes public and private sector funding for AIDS. Serves as a national information resource. Holds an annual conference. Operates a mail order pharmacy. Publishes newsletters "The Active Voice," "NAPWA Notes," and "Medical Alert." Newsletters plus information about pharmacy and daily medical alerts are available on the web site.

National Cancer Institute (NCI)
Physician Data Query (PDQ)
CancerNet
CANCERLIT
LiveHelp
31 Center Drive MSC 2580
Building 31, Room 10A03
Bethesda, MD 20892
(800) 422-6237   (800) 332-8615 (TT)   FAX (301) 402-5874
CancerFax (800) 624-2511   e-mail: cancermail@cips.nci.nih.gov
cancer.gov

The National Cancer Institute supports basic and clinical research investigations into the causes, prevention, and cure for cancer. The PDQ database provides up-to-date information on cancer prevention, screening, treatments, and care. PDQ is available on the Internet through CancerNet, which also contains fact sheets and publications, CancerNet news, and CANCERLIT abstracts and citations. CancerFax provides access by fax machine to information statements from the PDQ Database, CANCERLIT citations and abstracts, and fact sheets on cancer topics. LiveHelp is a pilot program that provides live, online assistance from an NCI Information Specialist; available Monday-Friday, 12-4 pm, Eastern Time. Most information is also available in Spanish. Calling the "800" phone number listed above connects with the regional center closest to you, which can provide information about the resources described above as well as local resources.

National Hospice and Palliative Care Organization (NHPCO)
1700 Diagonal Road, Suite 300
Alexandria, VA 22314
(800) 658-8898   (703) 837-1500   FAX (703) 525-5762
www.nho.org

A group that advocates for the rights of terminally ill patients and promotes hospice. Provides informational and educational materials and referrals. The web site enables users to locate hospices in their geographic area. For referral to a hospice, call NHPCO's toll-free Hospice Helpline at 800-658-8898. Offers three brochures, "Communicating Your End of Life Wishes," "How to Select a Hospice Program," and "The Medicare Hospice Benefit." Free. Also available on the web site.

Oncolink
University of Pennsylvania Cancer Center
www.oncolink.upenn.edu

This online resource enables users to search for cancer information by topic. It includes the data in Cancerlit and PDQ (see listing for National Cancer Institute). Videotapes on various topics are available on the web site.

Partnership for Caring
PO Box 97290
Washington, DC 20077-7205
(800) 989-9455   (202) 296-8071
FAX (202) 296-8352   e-mail: pfc@partnershipforcaring.org
www.partnershipforcaring.org

Provides advance directive forms (living will and medical power of attorney) tailored to individual state legal requirements; $5.00 per set. Advance directive forms may be downloaded from web site. Membership, $35.00, includes quarterly newsletter, "Choices."

Viatical and Life Settlement Association of America (VLSAA)
2025 M Street, NW, Suite 800
Washington, DC 20036
(800) 842-9811   (202) 367-1136   FAX (202) 367-2136
e-mail: VLSAA@dc.sba.com   www.viatical.org

The members of this trade association purchase life insurance policies owned by individuals who are terminally ill in return for a cash settlement. Referrals are made to association members. Also available on web site.

<u>The Wellness Community</u>
35 East 7th Street, Suite 412
Cincinnati, OH 45202
(513) 421-7111   FAX (513) 421-7119
e-mail: help@wellness-community.org
www.wellness-community.org

Provides free psychological, social, and educational support services for adults with cancer, their families, and friends as an adjunct to medical treatment. Affiliates are located across the country.

Advanced Breast Cancer: A Guide to Living with Metastatic Disease
by Musa Mayer
O'Reilly and Associates
101 Morris Street
Sebastopol, CA 95472
(800) 998-9938   (707) 829-0515
e-mail: order@oreilly.com   www.patientcenters.com

Although this book specifically discusses metastatic breast cancer, it applies to other types of metastatic cancer and terminal illness. It describes the shock of recurrence, treatment choices, pain relief, and the personal stories of patients and their families. Includes listings of organizations, publications, and online resources. $19.95 plus $4.50 shipping and handling

AIDS Care at Home
by Judith Greif and Beth Ann Golden
John Wiley and Sons
1 Wiley Drive
Somerset, NJ 08875
(800) 225-5945   (732) 469-4400   www.wiley.com

Written by two nurses who specialize in treating people with HIV/AIDS, this book provides practical information for caregivers on the daily needs of people with AIDS. Includes information on emotional stress, how to recognize the symptoms of diseases that affect people with AIDS, when to consult a physician, and resources for the various potential conditions. $17.95 plus $5.00 shipping and handling

Before I Die: Medical Care and Personal Choices
Films for the Humanities and Sciences
PO Box 2053
Princeton, NJ 08543
(800) 257-5126   FAX (609) 275-3767
e-mail: custserv@films.com   www.films.com

In this videotape, a panel discusses issues such as advance directives, physician-assisted suicide, and palliative care. Purchase, $129.00; rental, $75.00; plus 6% shipping and handling.

Caregiving - A Step-By-Step Resource for Caring for the Person with Cancer at Home
by Peter S. Houts and Julia A. Bucher
American Cancer Society (ACS)
NCICFUL
PO Box 102454
Atlanta, GA 30368
(800) 227-2345   www.cancer.org

This guide provides information about cancer treatments, managing care, emotional and physical conditions often associated with cancer, and living with cancer and cancer treatments. Includes resource list. $14.95

Caring for Yourself While Caring for Others: Survival and Renewal
by Lawrence M. Brammer
Vantage Press
516 West 34th Street
New York, NY 10001
(800) 882-3273   (212) 736-1767   FAX (212) 736-2273
www.vantagepress.com

This book discusses coping and survival strategies and suggests how to face difficult feelings. Provides community resources and reading lists. $14.95 plus $2.50 shipping and handling

Childhood Leukemia: A Guide for Families, Friends, and Caregivers
by Nancy Keene
O'Reilly and Associates
101 Morris Street
Sebastopol, CA 95472
(800) 998-9938   (707) 829-0515
e-mail: order@oreilly.com   www.patientcenters.com

In addition to basic information on caring for the child with leukemia, this book offers practical suggestions and emotional support during hospitalizations, chemotherapy and radiation treatment, relapse, death, and bereavement. Chapters include resource organizations and publications. $24.95 plus $4.50 shipping and handling

Controlling Cancer Pain: A Video for Patients and Families
Cancer Information Center, National Cancer Institute (NCI)
31 Center Drive MSC 2580
Building 31, Room 10A03
Bethesda, MD 20892
(800) 422-6237   (800) 332-8615 (TT)   FAX (301) 402-5874
CancerFax (800) 624-2511   e-mail: cancermail@cips.nci.nih.gov
cancer.gov

238

In this videotape, three individuals describe the pain management techniques they use. Includes oral and intravenous medications and patient controlled analgesia (PCA). Closed captioned. 12 minutes. Free

Dying At Home: A Family Guide for Caregiving
by Andrea Sankar
Johns Hopkins University Press
PO Box 50370
Baltimore, MD 21211-4370
(800) 537-5487   FAX (410) 516-6998   www.press.jhu.edu/press

Using extensive interviews with individuals, family members, and professional caregivers, this book discusses the decision to die at home. Offers practical suggestions for health care including nutrition, mobility, medication, and pain control. $16.95 plus $4.00 shipping and handling

Everyone's Guide to Cancer Therapy
by Malin Dollinger, Ernest H. Rosenbaum, and Greg Cable
Andrews and McMeel
PO Box 419150
Kansas City, MO 64141
(800) 642-6480

This book describes the diagnosis, treatment, and daily management of common cancers, including breast cancer. Includes chapters on treatment options, supportive care, sexuality, improving quality of life, and new advances in research, diagnosis and treatment. Provides a glossary of medical terms plus lists of anticancer drugs and their side effects, cancer associations and support groups, comprehensive cancer care centers, clinical trials sites, and suggested reading. $21.95 plus $4.25 shipping and handling

Facing Death
FEPI/Family Experiences Productions, Inc.
401 West 15th Street, Suite 680
Austin, TX 78701
(512) 494-0338   FAX (512) 494-0340
e-mail: fepi@texas.net   www.fepi.com/html/facing_death.html

There are four videotapes in this series. "Providing Physical, Emotional & Spiritual Comfort to Loved Ones" offers suggestions from caregivers, physicians, social workers, hospice professionals, and patients. 33 minutes. Individuals, $19.95: institutions, $59.95. "Practical Planning and Legal Issues" discusses end-of-life decisions. 17 minutes. Individuals, $16.95; institutions, $44.95. "Understanding End-of-Life Patient Needs" focuses on emotional issues. 15 minutes. Individuals, $19.95; institutions, $59.95. "The Gift of Being There" describes the importance of support from family and friends; 13 minutes; individuals, $19.95; institutions, $59.95; plus $6.50 shipping and handling for any number of tapes.

A Fate Worse than Death
Fanlight Productions
4196 Washington Street, Suite 2
Boston, MA 02131
(800) 937-4113   (617) 469-4999   FAX (617) 469-3379
e-mail: fanlight@fanlight.com   www.fanlight.com

This videotape follows family members as they decide whether to end the life support systems for a loved one. Also includes a discussion of living wills and durable powers of attorney. Purchase, $145.00; rent, $50.00 per day

Handbook for Mortals: Guidance for People Facing Serious Illness
by Joanne Lynn and Joan Harrold
Oxford University Press
2001 Evans Road
Cary, NC 27513
(800) 451-7556   FAX (919) 677-1303
e-mail: orders@oup-usa.org   www.oup-usa.org

This book examines issues of serious illness and dying such as caregiving, pain control, communicating with health professionals, treatment decisions, sudden death, death of a child, planning a funeral, and grieving. Includes resource list. $15.95

Home Care for Seriously Ill Children: A Manual for Parents
by Ida M. Martinson and D. Gay Moldow
Children's Hospice International
2202 Mt. Vernon Avenue, Suite 3C
Alexandria, VA 22301
(800) 242-4453   (703) 684-0330   FAX (703) 684-0226
e-mail: chiorg@aol.com   www.chionline.org

This manual provides guidance to parents who decide to care for children with life-threatening illnesses at home. $7.95 plus $3.50 shipping and handling

Home Care for the Critically and Terminally Ill
Life Concerns
PO Box 68255
Oro Valley, AZ 85737
(888) 266-3608   (520) 219-5952   FAX (561) 382-3953
e-mail: info@lifeconcerns.com   www.lifeconcerns.com

This six part video series, which follows a young man who is terminally ill, looks at caregiving from the caregiver's perspective. Provides practical information and emotional support. $200.00

Hospice Care for Children
by Ann Armstrong-Dailey and Sarah Zarbock Goltzer (eds.)
Children's Hospice International
2202 Mt. Vernon Avenue, Suite 3C
Alexandria, VA 22301
(800) 242-4453   (703) 684-0330   FAX (703) 684-0226
e-mail: chiorg@aol.com   www.chionline.org

A book that covers a variety of issues that affect children who are dying, including pain control, family dynamics, and home care. Includes list of children's literature on death. $45.00 plus $6.50 shipping and handling

The Hospice Movement: A Better Way of Caring for the Dying
by Sandol Stoddard
Random House

This book describes the history of hospice care as well as the various forms hospice care can take. It includes information about pain control. Out of print.

Informed Decisions: The Complete Book of Cancer Diagnosis, Treatment, and Recovery
by Gerald P. Murphy, Lois B. Morris, and Dianne Lange
American Cancer Society (ACS)
NCICFUL
PO Box 102454
Atlanta, GA 30368
(800) 227-2345   www.cancer.org

In addition to diagnosis and treatment, this book discusses coping strategies, pain control, advanced illness, and the special needs of children with cancer and AIDS-related cancers. Provides an encyclopedia of common and uncommon cancers. Includes listings of Comprehensive Cancer Centers, Clinical Cancer Centers, Clinical Trials Cooperative Groups, Community Clinical Oncology Programs, cancer registries, as well as online resources and patient education, support, and advocacy organizations. $29.95

Letting Go: A Hospice Journey
Films for the Humanities and Sciences
PO Box 2053
Princeton, NJ 08543
(800) 257-5126   FAX (609) 275-3767
e-mail: custserv@films.com   www.films.com

This film relates the hospice experiences of a young boy with incurable brain disease, a midlle-aged woman who has lung cancer, and an elder with a brain tumor and their families and the health care professionals and volunteers who provide the service. 90 minutes. Purchase, $149.00; rental, $75.00; plus 6% shipping and handling

Living with Life-Threatening Illness: A Guide for Patients, Their Families, & Caregivers
by Kenneth J. Doka
Jossey-Bass Inc.
350 Sansome Street, 5th floor
San Francisco, CA 94104
(800) 956-7739   (415) 433-1767   FAX (800) 605-2665
josseybass.com

This book discusses individuals' responses to life-threatening illness and coping with various phases of illness, the possibility of recovery, and the terminal phase. Includes effects on the family and special populations, such as children and elders, and makes suggestions for health professionals and caregivers. $28.00 plus $5.50 shipping and handling

The Measure of Our Days
by Jerome Groopman
Viking/Penguin Putnam
375 Hudson Street
New York, NY 10014
(800) 788-6262   www.penguinputnam.com

Written by a physician who cares for patients with cancer and AIDS, this book uses real cases to depict a humane type of medical care, where the physician is aware of the social aspects of his patients' lives. $13.95 plus $2.75 shipping and handling

Medicare Hospice Benefits: A Special Way of Caring for People Who Have a Terminal Illness
Centers for Medicare and Medicaid Services (CMS)
formerly Health Care Financing Administration (HCFA)
7500 Security Boulevard
Baltimore, MD 21244
(800) 633-4227   (410) 786-3000   www.hcfa.gov
www.medicare.gov

Discusses hospice care, eligibility requirements, and Medicare coverage. Free. Also available in large print. Also available on the web site.

On Death and Dying
by Elisabeth Kubler-Ross
Simon and Schuster
100 Front Street
Riverside, NJ 08075
(888) 866-6631   FAX (800) 943-9831   www.simonsays.com

This classic work written by a psychiatrist who specializes in end-of-life issues discusses the five stages that patients go through when they are terminally ill, effects on the family, and therapy. Hardcover, $23.00; softcover, $12.00; plus $4.98 shipping and handling.

On Our Own Terms: Moyers on Dying
Films for the Humanities and Sciences
PO Box 2053
Princeton, NJ 08543
(800) 257-5126   FAX (609) 275-3767
e-mail: custserv@films.com   www.films.com

This set of four videotapes explores the issues of death and dying, with host Bill Moyers. Includes "Living with Dying," "A Different Kind of Care," "A Death of One's Own," and "A Time to Change." Topics discussed include caregiving, pain management, advance directives, and discussing end of life decisions with loved ones. Each videotape, 87 minutes. Individuals, $99.95 plus $6.00 shipping and handling; institutions, $299.00 plus $17.95 shipping and handling. Discussion guide included.

Palliative Pain and Symptom Management for Children and Adolescents
by Robert A. Milch with Arnold Freeman and Ellen Clark
Children's Hospice International
2202 Mt. Vernon Avenue, Suite 3C
Alexandria, VA 22301
(800) 242-4453   (703) 684-0330   FAX (703) 684-0226
e-mail: chiorg@aol.com   www.chionline.org

This manual for health care providers describes strategies for management of acute and chronic pain in terminally ill children. $7.95 plus $3.50 shipping and handling

Parting Company: Understanding the Loss of a Loved One/The Caregiver's Journey
by Cynthia Pearson and Margaret L. Stubbs
Seal Press
3131 Western Avenue, Suite 410
Seattle, WA 98121
(800) 754-0271   (206) 283-7844   FAX (206) 285-9410
e-mail: sealprss@scn.org   www.sealpress.com

In this book, 14 caregivers share their experiences in caring for loved ones before they died. These survivors' perspectives provide vital details of the realities of end-of-life care. $18.95 plus $5.00 shipping and handling

Primer of Palliative Care
by Porter Storey
Kendall-Hunt Publishing
4050 Westmark Drive
PO Box 1840
Dubuque, IA 52004-1840
(800) 228-0810   (563) 589-1000   FAX (800) 772-9165
www.kendallhunt.com

This booklet, written by the medical director of a hospice, provides information on pain management as well as psychological, social, and spiritual needs of patients. $6.00 plus $5.00 shipping and handling

Teamwork: The Cancer Patient's Guide to Talking with Your Doctor
National Coalition for Cancer Survivorship (NCCS)
1010 Wayne Avenue, Suite 770
Silver Spring, MD 20910
(877) 622-7937   (301) 650-9127   FAX (301) 565-9670
e-mail: info@cansearch.org   www.cansearch.org

This publication provides practical suggestions to help people with cancer communicate with their doctors. Based on the experience of individuals with cancer, it includes questions you should ask and information the doctor should get from you. Available in English and Spanish. Free plus $2.00 shipping and handling

To Choose No Harm
Fanlight Productions
4196 Washington Street, Suite 2
Boston, MA 02131
(800) 937-4113   (617) 469-4999   FAX (617) 469-3379
e-mail: fanlight@fanlight.com   www.fanlight.com

This videotape presents discussions regarding medical decision-making at the end of life by professional caregivers, when conflict exists between the patients and professionals or patients and family members. The cases include a young man with AIDS and an older women with terminal cancer. 45 minutes. Purchase, $195.00; rental, $50.00 per day; plus $9.00 shipping and handling.

Understanding Cancer Pain
Cancer Information Center, National Cancer Institute (NCI)
31 Center Drive MSC 2580
Building 31, Room 10A03
Bethesda, MD 20892
(800) 422-6237   (800) 332-8615 (TT)   FAX (301) 402-5874
CancerFax (800) 624-2511   e-mail: cancermail@cips.nci.nih.gov
cancer.gov

This booklet describes methods used to control cancer pain and provides a pain rating scale and pain diary. Large print. Available in English and Spanish. Also available on the web site.

Viatical Settlements: A Guide for People with Terminal Illnesses
Federal Trade Commission
600 Pennsylvania Avenue, NW, Room H-130
Washington, DC 20580
(877) 382-4357   FAX (202) 326-2572
e-mail: publications@ftc.gov   www.ftc.gov

This brochure discusses the sale of a terminally ill individual's life insurance policy for a lump sum cash payment and provides consumer guidelines to those considering such settlements. Free. Also available on the web site.

INDEX OF ORGANIZATIONS

This index contains only those organizations listed under sections titled "ORGANI-ZATIONS" and "INTERNET RESOURCES." These organizations may also be listed as vendors of publications and tapes.

PUBLICATIONS FROM RESOURCES FOR REHABILITATION

Making Wise Medical Decisions
How to Get the Information You Need

This book includes a wealth of information about where to go and what to read in order to make informed, rational, medical decisions. It describes a plan for obtaining relevant health information, and evaluating the quality of medical tests and procedures, health care providers, and health facilities. Each chapter includes extensive resources to help the reader get started. Includes Internet resources.

Second edition, 2001   ISBN 0-929718-29-1 $42.95

*"It is **refreshing** to find a source of **practical information** on how to proceed through the medical maze...this should become a popular resource in any public, hospital, or academic library's consumer health collection."* **Library Journal**
*"The book is **very,very good**. There's so much information, it's **definitely worth buying**."* **A health care consumer**

The Mental Health Resource Guide

In a landmark report, the Surgeon General of the U.S. declared that mental illness is a public health problem of great magnitude. Both the public and professionals hold misconceptions about mental disorders. The Mental Health Resource Guide is designed to help individuals who are mentally ill, their family members, and health professionals understand the issues surrounding mental illness and find services and advocates who can help them. The book provides information on treatments in current use, medications, laws that affect individuals who are mentally ill, employment, and the needs of children and elders. The effects of mental illness on the family and caregivers are also addressed. Chapters on anxiety disorders, eating disorders, depressive disorders, schizophrenia, and addictions include information about causes, diagnoses, and treatments as well as descriptions of helpful organizations, publications, and tapes. Includes Internet resources.

2001   ISBN 0-929718-27-5 $39.95

*"...**authoritative**...will add **value** to professional health care collections and public libraries."* **Library Journal**

A Woman's Guide to Coping with Disability

This <u>unique</u> book addresses the special needs of women with disabilities and chronic conditions, such as social relationships, sexual functioning, pregnancy, childrearing, caregiving, and employment. Special attention is paid to ways in which women can advocate for their rights with the health care and rehabilitation systems. Written for women in all age categories, the book has chapters on the disabilities that are most prevalent in women or likely to affect the roles and physical functions unique to women. Included are arthritis, diabetes, epilepsy, lupus, multiple sclerosis, osteoporosis, and spinal cord injury. Each chapter also includes information about the condition, professional service providers, and psychological aspects plus descriptions of organizations, publications and tapes, and special assistive devices. Includes Internet resources.

Third edition, 2000   ISBN 0-929718-26-7 $44.95

*Chosen by **Library Journal** as a book of outstanding quality and significance.* *"...**this excellent, empowering** resource belongs in all collections."*
*"...**crucial information** women need to be informed, empowered, and in control of their lives. **Excellent** self-help information... **Highly recommended** for public and academic libraries."* **Choice**
*"...a **marvelous** publication...will help women feel more in control of their lives."* **A nurse who became disabled**

A Man's Guide to Coping with Disability

Written to fill the void in the literature regarding the special needs of men with disabilities, this book includes information about men's responses to disability, with a special emphasis on the values men place on independence, occupational achievement, and physical activity. Information on finding local services, self-help groups, laws that affect men with disabilities, sports and recreation, and employment is applicable to men with any type of disability or chronic condition. The disabilities that are most prevalent in men or that affect men's special roles in society are included. Chapters on coronary heart disease, diabetes, HIV/AIDS, multiple sclerosis, prostate conditions, spinal cord injury, and stroke include information about the disease or condition, psychological aspects, sexual functioning, where to find services, environmental adaptations, and annotated entries of organizations, publications and tapes, and resources for assistive devices. Includes Internet resources.

Second edition, 1999   ISBN 0-929718-23-2 $44.95

"a unique reference source." **Library Journal**
"a unique purchase for public libraries" **Booklist/Reference Books Bulletin**
"...Thank you for the **high quality** *books you provide."* **A nurse's aide**

Resources for People with Disabilities and Chronic Conditions

This comprehensive resource guide has chapters on spinal cord injury, low back pain, diabetes, multiple sclerosis, hearing and speech impairments, vision impairment and blindness, and epilepsy. Each chapter includes information about the disease or condition; psychological aspects of the condition; professional service providers; environmental adaptations; assistive devices; and descriptions of organizations, publications, and products. Chapters on rehabilitation services, independent living, self-help, laws that affect people with disabilities (including the ADA), and making everyday living easier. Special information for children is also included. Includes Internet resources.

Fourth edition, 1999   ISBN 0-929718-22-4 $54.95

"... **wide coverage** *and* **excellent** *organization of this encyclopedic guide...recommended..."* **Choice**
*"***Sensitive** *to the tremendous variety of needs and circumstances of living with a disability."*   **American Libraries**
"...an **excellent** *resource for consumers and professionals..."* **Journal of the American Paraplegia Society**
"...improves the chances of library patrons finding needed services..." **American Reference Books Annual**
"...an excellent reference that **should be in every family physician's office** *as well as in libraries..."*
Journal of the American Board of Family Physicians

Meeting the Needs of Employees with Disabilities

This resource guide provides the information people with disabilities need to retain or obtain employment. Includes information on government programs and laws such as the Americans with Disabilities Act, training programs, supported employment, transition from school to work, assistive technology, and environmental adaptations. Chapters on hearing and speech impairments, mobility impairments, and visual impairment and blindness describe organizations, adaptive equipment, and services plus suggestions for a safe and friendly workplace. Case vignettes describing accommodations for employees with disabilities are a special feature. Includes Internet resources.

Third edition, 1999   ISBN 0-929718-25-9 $44.95

"...an **excellent** *directory for those challenged with incorporating persons with disabilities in the workplace..."*
*"...***recommended** *for public libraries and for academic libraries..."* **Choice**

Resources for Elders with Disabilities

This book meets the needs of elders, family members, and other caregivers. Published in large print, the book provides information about rehabilitation, laws that affect elders with disabilities, and self-help groups. Each chapter that deals with a specific disability or condition has information on the causes and treatments for the condition; psychological aspects; professional service providers; where to find services; environmental adaptations; and suggestions for making everyday living safer and easier. Chapters on hearing loss, vision loss, Parkinson's disease, stroke, arthritis, osteoporosis, and diabetes also provide information on organizations, publications and tapes, and assistive devices. Throughout the book are practical suggestions to prevent accidents and to facilitate interactions with family members, friends, and service providers. Plus information about aids for everyday living, older workers, falls, travel, and housing. Includes Internet resources.

Fourth edition, 1999   ISBN 0-929718-24-0 $49.95

*"...especially useful for older readers. **Highly recommended.**" Library Journal*
*"...a **valuable, well organized, easy-to-read** reference source." American Reference Books Annual*
*"...a **handy ready-reference**..."   Reference Books Bulletin/Booklist*

Living with Low Vision: A Resource Guide for People with Sight Loss

This large print **(18 point bold type)** comprehensive guide helps people with sight loss locate the services, products, and publications that they need to keep reading, working, and enjoying life. Chapters for children and elders plus information on self-help groups, how to keep reading and working with vision loss, and making everyday living easier. Information on laws that affect people with vision loss, including the ADA, and high tech equipment that promotes independence and employment. Includes Internet resources.

Sixth edition, 2001   ISBN 0-929718-28-3 $46.95

*"No other complete resource guide exists..an **invaluable** tool for locating services.. for public and academic libraries."*
Library Journal
*"...a **very useful resource** for patients experiencing vision loss."   Archives of Ophthalmology*
*"...a **superb resource**...should be made available in waiting rooms or patient education areas..."*
American Journal of Ophthalmology
*"This volume is a **treasure chest** of concise, useful information."   OT Week*
*"...a **good reference** for libraries serving visually handicapped individuals."*
American Reference Books Annual

LARGE PRINT PUBLICATIONS
Designed for distribution by professionals to people with disabilities and chronic conditions

These publications serve as self-help guides for people with disabilities and chronic conditions. They include information on the condition, rehabilitation services, products, and resources that contribute to independence. Titles include **After a Stroke, Living with Diabetes, Living with Low Vision,** and **How to Keep Reading with Vision Loss.**

8 1/2" by 11"   Printed in **18 point bold type** on ivory paper with black ink for maximum contrast.

*"These are **exciting products**. We look forward to doing business with you again."   A rehabilitation professional*

Providing Services for People with Vision Loss: A Multidisciplinary Perspective
Susan L. Greenblatt, Editor

Written by ophthalmologists, rehabilitation professionals, a physician who has experienced vision loss, and a sociologist, this book discusses how various professionals can work together to provide coordinated care for people with vision loss. Chapters include Vision Loss: A Patient's Perspective; Vision Loss: An Ophthalmologist's Perspective; Operating a Low Vision Aids Service; The Need for Coordinated Care; Making Referrals for Rehabilitation Services; Mental Health Services: The Missing Link; Self-Help Groups for People with Sight Loss; and Aids and Techniques that Help People with Vision Loss plus a Glossary. Also available on cassette.

1989   ISBN 0-929718-02-X $19.95

*"...an **excellent** overview of the perspectives and clinical services that facilitate rehabilitation."*
Archives of Ophthalmology
*"...an **excellent** guide for professionals."*   **Journal of Rehabilitation**

Meeting the Needs of People with Vision Loss: A Multidisciplinary Perspective
Susan L. Greenblatt, Editor

Written by rehabilitation professionals, physicians, and a sociologist, this book discusses how to provide appropriate information and how to serve special populations. Chapters include What People with Vision Loss Need to Know; Information and Referral Services for People with Vision Loss; The Role of the Family in the Adjustment to Blindness or Visual Impairment; Diabetes and Vision Loss - Special Considerations; Special Needs of Children and Adolescents; Older Adults with Vision and Hearing Losses; Providing Services to Visually Impaired Elders in Long Term Care Facilities; plus a series of Multidisciplinary Case Studies. Also available on cassette.

1991   ISBN 0-929718-07-0 $24.95

"...of use to anyone concerned with improving service delivery to the growing population of people who are visually impaired."   **American Journal of Occupational Therapy**

See next page for order form.

RESOURCES for REHABILITATION →

33 Bedford Street, Suite 19A, Lexington, MA 02420
(781) 862-6455 FAX (781) 861-7517 e-mail: orders@rfr.org www.rfr.org
Our Federal Employer Identification Number is 04-2975-007

NAME _____

ORGANIZATION _____

ADDRESS _____

PHONE _____

[ ] Check or signed institutional purchase order enclosed for full amount of order. Purchase ord◄
accepted from government agencies, hospitals, and universities only.

[ ] Mastercard/VISA Card number: _____

Signature: _____Expiration date: _____

ALL ORDERS OF $100.00 OR LESS MUST BE PREPAID.

TITLE	QUANTITY	PRICE	TOTAL
Making Wise Medical Decisions	____ X	$42.95	_____
The Mental Health Resource Guide	____ X	39.95	_____
A Woman's Guide to Coping with Disability	____ X	44.95	_____
A Man's Guide to Coping with Disability	____ X	44.95	_____
Resources for People with Disabilities and Chronic Conditions	____ X	54.95	_____
Meeting the Needs of Employees with Disabilities	____ X	44.95	_____
Resources for Elders with Disabilities	____ X	49.95	_____
Living with Low Vision: A Resource Guide	____ X	46.95	_____
Providing Services for People with Vision Loss	____ X	19.95	_____
[ ] Check here for audiocassette edition			
Meeting the Needs of People with Vision Loss	____ X	24.95	_____
[ ] Check here for audiocassette edition			

MINIMUM PURCHASE OF 25 COPIES PER TITLE FOR THE FOLLOWING PUBLICATIONS
Call for discount on purchases of 100 or more copies of any single title.

After a stroke	____ X	1.75	_____
Living with diabetes	____ X	1.75	_____
Living with low vision	____ X	2.00	_____
How to keep reading with vision loss	____ X	1.75	_____
Living with age-related macular degeneration	____ X	1.25	_____
Aids for everyday living with vision loss	____ X	1.25	_____
Living with diabetic retinopathy	____ X	1.75	_____
High tech aids for people with vision loss	____ X	1.75	_____

SUB-TOTAL _____

SHIPPING & HANDLING: $50.00 or less, add $5.00; $50.01 to 100.00, add $8.00;
add $4.00 for each additional $100.00 or fraction of $100.00. Alaska, Hawaii,
U.S. territories, and Canada, add $3.00 to shipping and handling charges
Foreign orders must be prepaid in U.S. currency. Please write for shipping charges.

SHIPPING/HANDLING_____

Prices are subject to change.

TOTAL $_____